Introduction

Welcome to **"Diabetic Diet Cookbook After 50: 115+ A Culinary Guide to Managing Diabetes and Aging Gracefully."** This book is designed to be your trusted companion on the journey to better health, offering a wealth of recipes that cater specifically to the dietary needs and preferences of individuals over 50 who are managing diabetes.

As we age, maintaining a balanced and nutritious diet becomes increasingly crucial, especially for those living with diabetes. The right foods can help stabilize blood sugar levels, support overall well-being, and enhance quality of life. This cookbook is crafted with these principles in mind, combining delicious flavors with the nutritional balance necessary for managing diabetes effectively.

Within these pages, you will find over 115 carefully curated recipes that are not only easy to prepare but also delightful to the palate. Each recipe is designed to provide essential nutrients while keeping your blood sugar levels in check. Whether you are looking for hearty breakfasts, satisfying lunches, delightful dinners, or tempting snacks and desserts, this cookbook has something for every occasion and taste.

But this book offers more than just recipes. It is a comprehensive guide that provides practical tips for meal planning, grocery shopping, and understanding the nutritional needs specific to those over 50 with diabetes. You will also find insights into the importance of maintaining a healthy lifestyle, including regular physical activity and stress management techniques, to complement your dietary efforts.

Embark on this culinary journey with confidence, knowing that each recipe is a step towards better health and a more vibrant life. Let **"Diabetic Diet Cookbook After 50"** inspire you to create meals that not only nourish your body but also bring joy and satisfaction to your dining experience.

Here's to a delicious and healthful adventure in managing diabetes and aging gracefully!

1. Greek Yogurt with Berries and Nuts

Ingredient:

- 1 cup plain Greek yogurt (full•fat or low•fat)
- 1/2 cup mixed berries (such as blueberries, raspberries, blackberries)
- 2 tbsp chopped walnuts or almonds
- 1 tsp honey (optional)

Instructions:

1. In a bowl, place the Greek yogurt.

2. Top the yogurt with the mixed berries.

3. Sprinkle the chopped nuts over the top.

4. If desired, drizzle 1 tsp of honey over the top for a touch of sweetness.

Nutritional Information (per serving):
- Calories: 200
- Total Carbs: 15g
- Fiber: 4g
- Net Carbs: 11g
- Protein: 15g
- Fat: 10g

This recipe is a great option for a diabetic•friendly breakfast or snack. The Greek yogurt provides protein and probiotics, the berries add fiber and antioxidants, and the nuts offer healthy fats and additional nutrients. The carb count is moderate and the fiber helps slow the absorption of sugars. Feel free to adjust the amounts of each ingredient to suit your personal preferences and dietary needs.

2. Vegetable Omelette with Spinach and Mushrooms

Ingredient:

• 3 eggs
• 2 tbsp milk or water
• 1 tbsp butter or oil
• 1/2 cup sliced mushrooms
• 1 cup fresh spinach leaves, chopped
• 1/4 cup diced bell pepper (optional)
• 2 tbsp grated cheese (cheddar, feta, etc.)
• Salt and pepper to taste

Instructions:

1. Crack the eggs into a bowl, add the milk or water, and whisk together until well combined.

2. Heat a non•stick skillet over medium heat and melt the butter or heat the oil.

3. Add the mushrooms and sauté for 2•3 minutes until softened.

4. Add the spinach and bell pepper (if using) and cook for 1•2 minutes until the spinach is wilted.

5. Pour the egg mixture into the skillet and let it sit for 30 seconds to a minute to set the bottom.

6. Using a spatula, gently push the cooked egg from the edges into the center, tilting the pan to allow the uncooked egg to flow to the edges.

7. When the eggs are mostly set but still a bit runny on top, sprinkle the grated cheese over half of the omelette.

8. Fold the plain half of the omelette over the cheese half and slide onto a plate.

9. Season with salt and pepper to taste. Serve hot.

Enjoy your delicious vegetable•packed omelette!

3. Oatmeal with Chia Seeds and Fresh Fruit

Ingredient:

- 1/2 cup old·fashioned rolled oats
- 1 cup unsweetened almond milk (or low·fat dairy milk)
- 1 tbsp chia seeds
- 1/2 cup mixed fresh berries (such as blueberries, raspberries, blackberries)
- 1 tsp honey or maple syrup (optional)
- Cinnamon to taste

Instructions:

1. In a small saucepan, combine the rolled oats and almond milk. Bring to a simmer over medium heat, stirring occasionally.

2. Once the oats have thickened to your desired consistency, about 5·7 minutes, remove from heat.

3. Stir in the chia seeds and let sit for 2·3 minutes to allow the chia seeds to absorb some of the liquid.

4. Top the oatmeal with the fresh berries.

5. If desired, drizzle with a small amount of honey or maple syrup to add a touch of sweetness.

6. Sprinkle with cinnamon.

Tips for a Diabetic Diet After 50:

- Oats are a great source of fiber, which can help regulate blood sugar levels.
- Chia seeds are high in fiber, protein and omega·3s, all beneficial for diabetes management.
- Fresh berries are low in sugar and high in antioxidants.
- Use unsweetened almond milk or low·fat dairy milk to keep the carb and calorie count down.
- Limit added sweeteners like honey or maple syrup, using just a small drizzle if needed.
- Cinnamon may help improve insulin sensitivity.

This balanced breakfast provides fiber, protein, healthy fats and nutrients to help keep blood sugar stable throughout the morning.

4. Avocado and Tomato on Whole Grain Toast

Ingredient:

• 2 slices of whole grain or sprouted bread
• 1/2 ripe avocado, mashed
• 1 medium tomato, sliced
• 1 tbsp olive oil
• 1 tsp lemon juice
• Salt and pepper to taste
• Optional: 1 tbsp crumbled feta or goat cheese

Instructions:

1. Toast the whole grain or sprouted bread until lightly golden.

2. In a small bowl, mash the avocado with the olive oil and lemon juice until smooth.

3. Spread the mashed avocado evenly over the toasted bread slices.

4. Arrange the sliced tomatoes on top of the avocado.

5. Sprinkle with a pinch of salt and freshly ground black pepper.

6. If desired, crumble the feta or goat cheese over the top.

Tips for a Diabetic Diet After 50:

• Whole grain or sprouted bread is higher in fiber and lower in refined carbs compared to white bread.
• Avocado is a great source of healthy monounsaturated fats, which can help regulate blood sugar levels.
• Tomatoes are low in carbs and high in vitamins, minerals and antioxidants.
• Olive oil provides heart•healthy fats.
• Lemon juice adds a touch of acidity without adding sugar.
• Feta or goat cheese can provide a boost of protein.

This open•faced toast makes for a nutritious and satisfying breakfast or snack that is diabetic•friendly. The combination of healthy fats, fiber, and low•glycemic ingredients can help manage blood sugar levels.

5. Smoothie with Kale, Almond Milk, and Berries

Ingredient:

- 1 cup unsweetened almond milk
- 1 cup fresh kale, stems removed
- 1/2 cup mixed berries (such as blueberries, raspberries, blackberries)
- 1 tbsp chia seeds
- 1 tbsp almond butter
- 1 tsp honey (optional)

Instructions:

1. Add the almond milk, kale, berries, chia seeds, and almond butter to a high•powered blender.

2. Blend on high speed until the mixture is smooth and creamy, about 1•2 minutes.

3. Taste and add a teaspoon of honey if desired, for a touch of sweetness.

4. Pour the smoothie into a glass and enjoy immediately.

Tips for a Diabetic Diet After 50:

- Kale is a nutrient•dense leafy green that is low in carbs and high in fiber, vitamins, and minerals.
- Almond milk is a great dairy•free option that is low in carbs and calories compared to regular milk.
- Berries are a low•glycemic fruit, meaning they won't spike blood sugar levels as much as other fruits.
- Chia seeds are high in fiber, protein, and omega•3s, which can help regulate blood sugar.
- Almond butter provides healthy fats and a creamy texture without added sugars.
- Use just a small amount of honey if needed, as it still contains carbs.

This smoothie is packed with fiber, protein, healthy fats, and essential vitamins and minerals to support overall health and blood sugar management for those with diabetes after 50. The combination of kale, berries, and almond•based ingredients makes it a nutrient•dense and diabetic•friendly option.

6. Cottage Cheese with Pineapple

Ingredient:

• 1 cup low•fat or non•fat cottage cheese
• 1/2 cup fresh pineapple chunks
• 1 tsp honey (optional)
• Cinnamon to taste

Instructions:

1. Scoop the cottage cheese into a bowl or container.

2. Top the cottage cheese with the fresh pineapple chunks.

3. If desired, drizzle a small amount of honey over the top (about 1 tsp).

4. Sprinkle cinnamon over the top to taste.

Tips for a Diabetic Diet After 50:

• Cottage cheese is a great source of protein, which can help stabilize blood sugar levels.
• Pineapple is a lower•glycemic fruit, meaning it won't spike blood sugar as much as some other fruits.
• Use only a small amount of honey, if any, as it still contains carbs and sugar.
• Cinnamon may help improve insulin sensitivity and regulate blood sugar.

This simple snack or light meal provides a balance of protein, fiber, and natural sweetness from the pineapple. The cottage cheese adds creaminess and more protein to help keep you feeling full and satisfied.

For a diabetic diet after 50, this cottage cheese and pineapple dish is a nutritious and blood sugar•friendly option. The combination of nutrients can help manage blood sugar levels and support overall health.

7. Almond Flour Pancakes with Blueberries

Ingredient:

- 1 cup almond flour
- 2 eggs
- 1/4 cup unsweetened almond milk
- 1 tsp baking powder
- 1/4 tsp ground cinnamon
- 1/4 tsp vanilla extract
- 1 cup fresh or frozen blueberries
- 1•2 tsp butter or coconut oil for cooking

Instructions:

1. In a medium bowl, whisk together the almond flour, eggs, almond milk, baking powder, cinnamon, and vanilla extract until a smooth batter forms.

2. Gently fold in the blueberries.

3. Heat a non•stick skillet or griddle over medium heat and melt a small amount of butter or coconut oil.

4. Scoop the batter onto the hot surface, using about 1/4 cup per pancake.

5. Cook for 2•3 minutes per side, or until golden brown.

6. Serve the almond flour pancakes warm, with additional blueberries on top if desired.

Tips for a Diabetic Diet After 50:

- Almond flour is low in carbs and high in healthy fats and protein, making it a great alternative to traditional wheat flour.
- Eggs provide protein to help stabilize blood sugar levels.
- Unsweetened almond milk is low in carbs and calories compared to regular milk.
- Blueberries are a low•glycemic fruit, rich in antioxidants and fiber.
- Cinnamon may help improve insulin sensitivity.
- Avoid using maple syrup or other high•sugar toppings. Instead, enjoy the pancakes as•is or with a small amount of butter or nut butter.

These almond flour pancakes are a delicious and diabetes•friendly breakfast option. The combination of almond flour, eggs, and blueberries provides a nutrient•dense meal that can help manage blood sugar levels for those with diabetes after 50.

8. Chia Pudding with Almond Milk and Raspberries

Ingredient:

• 1/4 cup chia seeds
• 1 cup unsweetened almond milk
• 1 tsp vanilla extract
• 1/2 tsp ground cinnamon
• 1 tbsp honey or maple syrup (optional)
• 1 cup fresh or frozen raspberries

Instructions:

1. In a medium bowl, whisk together the chia seeds, almond milk, vanilla extract, and cinnamon until well combined.

2. Cover the bowl and refrigerate for at least 2 hours, or overnight, stirring occasionally, until the chia seeds have thickened the mixture into a pudding•like consistency.

3. If using honey or maple syrup, stir it in after the chia pudding has thickened.

4. Divide the chia pudding into serving bowls or jars.

5. Top each serving with 1/4 cup of fresh or frozen raspberries.

Tips for a Diabetic Diet:

• Chia seeds are high in fiber, protein, and omega•3s, which can help regulate blood sugar levels.
• Unsweetened almond milk is low in carbs and calories compared to dairy milk.
• Raspberries are a low•glycemic fruit, meaning they won't spike blood sugar levels.
• Use just a small amount of honey or maple syrup if needed, as these sweeteners still contain carbs.
• Cinnamon may help improve insulin sensitivity.

This chia pudding makes for a satisfying, nutrient•dense breakfast or snack that is perfect for a diabetic diet. The combination of chia, almond milk, and raspberries provides a delicious and blood sugar•friendly treat.

9. Scrambled Eggs with Bell Peppers and Onions

Ingredient:

• 3 large eggs
• 1 tbsp olive oil
• 1/4 cup diced bell pepper (any color)
• 1/4 cup diced onion
• 1 tbsp water or unsweetened almond milk
• Salt and pepper to taste
• Optional: 1 tbsp grated cheddar or feta cheese

Instructions:

1. In a small bowl, whisk the eggs together with the water or almond milk. Season with a pinch of salt and pepper.

2. Heat the olive oil in a non•stick skillet over medium heat. Add the diced bell pepper and onion. Sauté for 3•4 minutes until the vegetables are softened.

3. Pour the whisked eggs into the skillet with the vegetables. Use a spatula to gently push and fold the eggs as they cook, creating soft, fluffy curds.

4. Continue cooking the eggs, stirring occasionally, until they are fully cooked through but still moist, about 2•3 minutes total.

5. If using, sprinkle the grated cheese over the top of the scrambled eggs during the last 30 seconds of cooking. Serve the scrambled eggs hot.

Tips for a Diabetic Diet After 50:

• Eggs are an excellent source of protein, which can help stabilize blood sugar levels.
• Bell peppers and onions add fiber, vitamins, and minerals without significantly increasing carbs.
• Using a small amount of olive oil provides healthy fats.
• Almond milk is a low•carb, dairy•free alternative to regular milk.
• Cheese can add extra protein, but use it sparingly as it does contain some fat and calories.
• This dish is a simple, nutrient•dense breakfast that is well•suited for a diabetic diet.

These scrambled eggs with bell peppers and onions make for a filling and diabetes•friendly meal to start the day. The combination of protein, fiber, and healthy fats can help manage blood sugar levels for those with diabetes after 50.

10. Whole Grain English Muffin with Peanut Butter

Ingredient:

• 1 whole grain English muffin
• 2 tbsp natural peanut butter (no added sugar)
• 1 tsp chia seeds (optional)
• Cinnamon to taste

Instructions:

1. Toast the whole grain English muffin until lightly golden brown.

2. Spread the natural peanut butter evenly over the two muffin halves.

3. If desired, sprinkle the chia seeds over the peanut butter.

4. Lightly dust the top with ground cinnamon.

Tips for a Diabetic Diet After 50:

• Whole grain English muffins are higher in fiber and lower in refined carbs compared to white bread.
• Natural peanut butter is a great source of protein and healthy fats to help stabilize blood sugar levels.
• Chia seeds add extra fiber, protein, and omega•3s to help manage diabetes.
• Cinnamon may help improve insulin sensitivity and regulate blood sugar.
• Avoid using jelly, jam, or other high•sugar toppings. The peanut butter provides enough natural sweetness.

This simple breakfast or snack option provides a balance of complex carbs, protein, and healthy fats to help keep blood sugar stable throughout the morning. The whole grain muffin, peanut butter, and optional chia seeds and cinnamon make it a diabetes•friendly choice.

For those with diabetes after 50, this whole grain English muffin with peanut butter is a nutritious and satisfying way to start the day or curb hunger between meals.

11. Pumpkin Spice Overnight Oats

Ingredient:

- 1/2 cup old•fashioned rolled oats
- 1/2 cup unsweetened almond milk
- 2 tbsp canned pumpkin puree
- 1 tsp chia seeds
- 1/2 tsp pumpkin pie spice
- 1/2 tsp vanilla extract
- 1 tsp maple syrup (optional)
- Pinch of salt

Instructions:

1. In a medium•sized bowl or jar with a lid, combine the rolled oats, almond milk, pumpkin puree, chia seeds, pumpkin pie spice, vanilla extract, and a pinch of salt. Stir well to mix.

2. If using, drizzle the maple syrup over the top and stir again to incorporate.

3. Cover the bowl or jar and refrigerate overnight, or for at least 4 hours.

4. In the morning, give the overnight oats a good stir. The chia seeds and oats will have thickened the mixture.

5. Enjoy the pumpkin spice overnight oats chilled or at room temperature.

Tips for a Diabetic Diet After 50:

- Rolled oats are a complex carb that can help regulate blood sugar levels.
- Unsweetened almond milk is low in carbs and calories compared to dairy milk.
- Pumpkin puree is low in carbs and high in fiber, vitamins, and antioxidants.
- Chia seeds add extra fiber, protein, and omega•3s to help manage diabetes.
- Pumpkin pie spice provides flavor without added sugars.
- Use just a small amount of maple syrup, if desired, as it still contains carbs.

This pumpkin spice overnight oats recipe is a delicious and diabetes•friendly breakfast option. The combination of complex carbs, fiber, protein, and healthy fats can help stabilize blood sugar levels and keep you feeling full and satisfied throughout the morning.

12. Low•Carb Breakfast Burrito with Turkey Sausage

Ingredient:

• 2 eggs, scrambled
• 2 oz cooked turkey sausage, crumbled
• 1/4 cup diced bell pepper
• 1/4 cup diced onion
• 1 tbsp olive oil
• 1 low•carb or whole wheat tortilla
• 1 oz shredded cheddar cheese
• Salt and pepper to taste

Instructions:

1. In a skillet, heat the olive oil over medium heat. Add the diced bell pepper and onion and sauté for 3•4 minutes until softened.

2. Add the crumbled turkey sausage to the skillet and cook for an additional 2•3 minutes, stirring occasionally.

3. Pour the scrambled eggs into the skillet and gently fold everything together until the eggs are cooked through.

4. Season the egg mixture with salt and pepper to taste.

5. Lay the low•carb or whole wheat tortilla on a flat surface. Spoon the egg, sausage, and vegetable mixture onto the center of the tortilla.

6. Sprinkle the shredded cheddar cheese over the top. Fold the bottom of the tortilla up, then fold in the sides and roll up tightly to create a burrito.

Tips for a Diabetic Diet After 50:

• Turkey sausage is a leaner protein option compared to pork sausage.
• Eggs provide protein and nutrients to help stabilize blood sugar levels.
• Bell peppers and onions add fiber, vitamins, and minerals without significantly increasing carbs.
• Using a low•carb or whole wheat tortilla helps keep the carb count down.
• Cheddar cheese provides additional protein and healthy fats.
• This breakfast burrito is a balanced meal with protein, fiber, and healthy fats to help manage blood sugar throughout the morning.

13. Smoked Salmon and Cream Cheese on Whole Grain Bagel

Ingredient:

- 1 whole grain bagel, toasted
- 2 tbsp reduced·fat cream cheese
- 2 oz smoked salmon
- 1 tbsp thinly sliced red onion (optional)
- 1 tbsp capers (optional)
- Freshly ground black pepper

Instructions:

1. Toast the whole grain bagel until lightly golden.

2. Spread the reduced·fat cream cheese evenly over the toasted bagel halves.

3. Top each bagel half with 1 oz of smoked salmon.

4. If desired, add a few thin slices of red onion and a sprinkle of capers.

5. Finish by grinding some black pepper over the top.

Tips for a Diabetic Diet After 50:

- Whole grain bagels are higher in fiber and lower in refined carbs compared to white bagels.
- Reduced·fat cream cheese provides protein and healthy fats without as much saturated fat.
- Smoked salmon is an excellent source of protein and omega·3 fatty acids, which can help manage diabetes.
- Red onion and capers add flavor without significantly increasing carbs.
- Avoid adding any additional sweeteners or high·sugar toppings.

This open·faced smoked salmon and cream cheese bagel is a nutrient·dense and diabetes·friendly breakfast or snack option. The combination of complex carbs, protein, and healthy fats can help stabilize blood sugar levels and keep you feeling full and satisfied.

For those with diabetes after 50, this whole grain bagel with smoked salmon and cream cheese makes for a delicious and blood sugar·friendly meal.

14. Mushroom and Swiss Cheese Frittata

Ingredient:

• 6 large eggs
• 1/4 cup unsweetened almond milk
• 1 tbsp olive oil
• 8 oz sliced mushrooms
• 1/2 cup diced onion
• 2 cloves garlic, minced
• 1/2 cup shredded Swiss cheese
• Salt and pepper to taste

Instructions:

1. Preheat your oven to 375°F.

2. In a medium bowl, whisk together the eggs and almond milk. Season with a pinch of salt and pepper.

3. Heat the olive oil in a 9•inch oven•safe non•stick skillet over medium heat. Add the sliced mushrooms and diced onion. Sauté for 5•7 minutes, until the vegetables are softened.

4. Add the minced garlic and cook for an additional 1 minute, until fragrant.

5. Pour the egg mixture over the sautéed vegetables in the skillet. Sprinkle the shredded Swiss cheese evenly over the top.

6. Transfer the skillet to the preheated oven and bake for 15•18 minutes, until the frittata is set and the cheese is melted. Remove the frittata from the oven and let it cool for 5 minutes before slicing and serving.

Tips for a Diabetic Diet After 50:

• Eggs are an excellent source of protein, which can help stabilize blood sugar levels.
• Mushrooms are low in carbs and provide fiber, vitamins, and minerals.
• Swiss cheese is a good source of protein and healthy fats.
• Almond milk is a low•carb, dairy•free alternative to regular milk.
• This frittata is a one•pan meal that provides a balance of protein, healthy fats, and fiber to help manage diabetes.
• Serve the frittata with a side salad or roasted vegetables for a complete, diabetes•friendly meal.

15. Quinoa Breakfast Bowl with Almonds and Cranberries

Ingredient:

- 1/2 cup cooked quinoa, cooled
- 1/2 cup unsweetened almond milk
- 2 tbsp sliced almonds
- 2 tbsp dried cranberries
- 1 tsp honey (optional)
- 1/4 tsp ground cinnamon

Instructions:

1. In a bowl, combine the cooked quinoa and almond milk. Stir to mix well.

2. Top the quinoa mixture with the sliced almonds and dried cranberries.

3. If desired, drizzle a small amount of honey (about 1 tsp) over the top.

4. Sprinkle the ground cinnamon over the bowl.

Tips for a Diabetic Diet After 50:

- Quinoa is a whole grain that is high in fiber, protein, and complex carbs, making it a great choice for managing blood sugar levels.

- Unsweetened almond milk is low in carbs and calories compared to dairy milk.

- Almonds provide healthy fats, fiber, and protein to help keep you feeling full and satisfied.

- Dried cranberries are a lower•glycemic fruit option, but use them in moderation as they still contain natural sugars.

- Cinnamon may help improve insulin sensitivity and regulate blood sugar.

- Use just a small amount of honey, if any, as it still contains carbs and sugar.

This quinoa breakfast bowl is a nutrient•dense and diabetes•friendly option. The combination of complex carbs, protein, healthy fats, and fiber can help stabilize blood sugar levels and provide sustained energy throughout the morning. It's a great way to start the day for those with diabetes after 50.

16. Grilled Chicken Salad with Mixed Greens and Vinaigrette

Ingredient:

• 4 oz grilled chicken breast, sliced
• 4 cups mixed greens (such as spinach, arugula, kale)
• 1/2 cup cherry tomatoes, halved
• 1/4 cup sliced cucumber
• 2 tbsp sliced almonds
• 2 tbsp crumbled feta cheese
• 2 tbsp olive oil
• 1 tbsp balsamic vinegar
• 1 tsp Dijon mustard
• 1 tsp lemon juice
• Salt and pepper to taste

Instructions:

1. In a large salad bowl, combine the mixed greens, cherry tomatoes, cucumber, sliced almonds, and crumbled feta cheese.

2. In a small bowl, whisk together the olive oil, balsamic vinegar, Dijon mustard, and lemon juice. Season with a pinch of salt and pepper.

3. Add the grilled chicken slices to the salad.

4. Drizzle the vinaigrette over the salad and toss gently to coat.

Tips for a Diabetic Diet After 50:

• Grilled chicken is a lean protein that can help stabilize blood sugar levels.
• Mixed greens are low in carbs and high in fiber, vitamins, and minerals.
• Cherry tomatoes and cucumber add additional nutrients without significantly increasing carbs.
• Sliced almonds provide healthy fats and a crunchy texture.
• Feta cheese adds protein and healthy fats.
• The olive oil and balsamic vinegar•based vinaigrette is a diabetes•friendly dressing, providing healthy fats without added sugars.

This grilled chicken salad with mixed greens and a simple vinaigrette is a nutritious and satisfying meal option for those following a diabetic diet after 50. The combination of lean protein, non•starchy vegetables, and healthy fats can help manage blood sugar levels.

17. Quinoa Salad with Chickpeas and Veggies

Ingredient:

• 1 cup cooked quinoa, cooled
• 1 (15 oz) can chickpeas, rinsed and drained
• 1 cup diced cucumber
• 1 cup cherry tomatoes, halved
• 1/2 cup diced red onion
• 1/2 cup crumbled feta cheese
• 2 tbsp chopped fresh parsley
• 2 tbsp olive oil
• 1 tbsp red wine vinegar
• 1 tsp Dijon mustard
• 1 tsp honey (optional)
• Salt and pepper to taste

Instructions:

1. In a large bowl, combine the cooked quinoa, chickpeas, cucumber, cherry tomatoes, red onion, feta cheese, and parsley.

2. In a small bowl, whisk together the olive oil, red wine vinegar, Dijon mustard, and honey (if using). Season with a pinch of salt and pepper.

3. Pour the dressing over the quinoa salad and toss gently to coat.

4. Refrigerate the salad for at least 30 minutes to allow the flavors to meld.

5. Serve chilled or at room temperature.

Tips for a Diabetic Diet After 50:

• Quinoa is a high•fiber, high•protein grain that can help regulate blood sugar levels.
• Chickpeas are a good source of fiber, protein, and complex carbs.
• Vegetables like cucumber, tomatoes, and onion add fiber, vitamins, and minerals without significantly increasing carbs.
• Feta cheese provides protein and healthy fats.
• The olive oil and vinegar dressing adds healthy fats without added sugars.
• Use just a small amount of honey, if desired, as it still contains carbs.

This quinoa salad with chickpeas and veggies is a nutrient•dense and diabetes•friendly option. The combination of complex carbs, protein, fiber, and healthy fats can help manage blood sugar levels for those with diabetes after 50.

18. Turkey and Avocado Wrap with Whole Grain Tortilla

Ingredient:

• 1 whole grain tortilla or wrap
• 3 oz sliced turkey breast
• 1/2 avocado, sliced
• 1/4 cup shredded lettuce
• 1 tbsp plain Greek yogurt
• 1 tsp Dijon mustard
• Salt and pepper to taste

Instructions:

1. Lay the whole grain tortilla or wrap on a flat surface.

2. Layer the sliced turkey breast evenly over the center of the tortilla.

3. Top the turkey with the sliced avocado and shredded lettuce.

4. In a small bowl, mix together the Greek yogurt and Dijon mustard. Spread this mixture over the avocado and lettuce.

5. Season with a pinch of salt and pepper.

6. Fold the bottom of the tortilla up, then fold in the sides and roll up tightly to create a wrap.

Tips for a Diabetic Diet After 50:

• Whole grain tortillas are higher in fiber and lower in refined carbs compared to white tortillas.
• Turkey breast is a lean protein that can help stabilize blood sugar levels.
• Avocado provides healthy monounsaturated fats, which can also help manage diabetes.
• Lettuce adds fiber and nutrients without significantly increasing carbs.
• Greek yogurt provides protein and a creamy texture, while the Dijon mustard adds flavor without added sugars.

This turkey and avocado wrap with a whole grain tortilla is a balanced, diabetes•friendly meal or snack. The combination of lean protein, healthy fats, and fiber can help keep blood sugar stable throughout the day for those with diabetes after 50.

19. Vegetable Stir•Fry with Tofu

Ingredient:

- 1 block (14 oz) extra•firm tofu, cubed
- 2 tbsp sesame oil
- 2 cups mixed vegetables (such as broccoli, bell peppers, snap peas, mushrooms)
- 1 clove garlic, minced
- 1 tsp grated fresh ginger
- 2 tbsp low•sodium soy sauce or tamari
- 1 tsp rice vinegar
- 1 tsp sesame seeds (optional)
- Salt and pepper to taste

Instructions:

1. Press the tofu block between paper towels or a clean kitchen towel to remove excess moisture. Cut the tofu into 1•inch cubes.

2. Heat the sesame oil in a large skillet or wok over medium•high heat. Add the tofu cubes and cook, stirring occasionally, until lightly browned on all sides, about 5•7 minutes. Transfer the tofu to a plate.

3. Add the mixed vegetables to the skillet. Stir•fry for 3•4 minutes, until the vegetables are crisp•tender.

4. Add the minced garlic and grated ginger to the skillet. Cook for 1 minute, until fragrant.

5. Return the cooked tofu to the skillet. Pour in the soy sauce and rice vinegar. Toss everything together until well combined and heated through.

6. Sprinkle the sesame seeds over the top, if using. Season with salt and pepper to taste. Serve the vegetable stir•fry with tofu immediately, over steamed brown rice or quinoa if desired.

Tips for a Diabetic Diet:

- Tofu is a great source of plant•based protein that won't spike blood sugar.
- Vegetables like broccoli, peppers, and mushrooms are low in carbs and high in fiber.
- Sesame oil and sesame seeds provide healthy fats.
- Soy sauce and rice vinegar add flavor without added sugars.
- This dish is a balanced meal with protein, fiber, and healthy fats to help manage diabetes.

20. Lentil Soup with Spinach and Carrots

Ingredient:

• 1 cup dry brown or green lentils, rinsed
• 4 cups low•sodium vegetable or chicken broth
• 1 tbsp olive oil
• 1 onion, diced
• 2 carrots, peeled and diced
• 2 cloves garlic, minced
• 1 tsp ground cumin
• 1 tsp dried oregano
• 1/4 tsp red pepper flakes (optional)
• 2 cups fresh spinach, chopped
• Salt and pepper to taste

Instructions:

1. In a large pot, combine the rinsed lentils and broth. Bring to a boil over high heat.
2. Reduce heat to medium•low, cover, and simmer for 15•20 minutes, until lentils are tender.
3. In a separate skillet, heat the olive oil over medium heat. Add the onion and carrots and sauté for 5•7 minutes, until softened.
4. Add the garlic, cumin, oregano, and red pepper flakes (if using). Cook for 1 minute, until fragrant.
5. Transfer the sautéed vegetables to the pot with the cooked lentils. Stir to combine.
6. Add the chopped spinach and cook for 2•3 minutes, until the spinach is wilted.
7. Season with salt and pepper to taste.

Tips for a Diabetic Diet After 50:

• Lentils are a great source of fiber, protein, and complex carbs, which can help regulate blood sugar levels.
• Spinach is a nutrient•dense leafy green that is low in carbs and high in vitamins and minerals.
• Carrots provide fiber, vitamins, and a natural sweetness without spiking blood sugar.
• Spices like cumin and oregano add flavor without added sugars or sodium.
• Using low•sodium broth helps control sodium intake, which is important for those with diabetes.
• This soup is a filling, nutrient•rich meal that can be enjoyed as the main course or as a side dish.

This lentil soup with spinach and carrots is an excellent option for a diabetic diet after 50, providing a balance of fiber, protein, and complex carbs to help manage blood sugar levels.

21. Grilled Salmon Caesar Salad

Ingredient:

- 4 oz grilled salmon fillet
- 4 cups chopped romaine lettuce
- 2 tbsp grated Parmesan cheese
- 2 tbsp low•fat Caesar dressing
- 1 tbsp toasted sliced almonds
- 1 tbsp whole wheat croutons (optional)
- Lemon wedge for serving

Instructions:

1. Grill or bake the salmon fillet until cooked through and flaky. Allow to cool slightly, then break into large flakes.

2. In a large salad bowl, combine the chopped romaine lettuce, grilled salmon flakes, Parmesan cheese, and low•fat Caesar dressing. Toss gently to coat.

3. Top the salad with the toasted sliced almonds and whole wheat croutons (if using).

4. Serve the Grilled Salmon Caesar Salad immediately, with a lemon wedge on the side.

Tips for a Diabetic Diet After 50:

- Salmon is an excellent source of protein and healthy omega•3 fatty acids, which can help regulate blood sugar levels.
- Romaine lettuce is a nutrient•dense leafy green that is low in carbs and high in fiber.
- Parmesan cheese provides protein and healthy fats without significantly increasing carbs.
- Low•fat Caesar dressing is a diabetes•friendly alternative to traditional creamy dressings.
- Toasted sliced almonds add a crunchy texture and healthy fats.
- Whole wheat croutons can be included for a bit of added fiber, but they are optional.

This Grilled Salmon Caesar Salad is a balanced and diabetes•friendly meal that combines lean protein, non•starchy vegetables, and healthy fats. The combination of nutrients can help manage blood sugar levels for those with diabetes after 50.

22. Stuffed Zucchini Boats with Ground Turkey

Ingredient:

• 4 medium zucchini, halved lengthwise
• 1 lb ground turkey
• 1 small onion, diced
• 2 cloves garlic, minced
• 1 cup diced tomatoes
• 1/2 cup shredded mozzarella cheese
• 2 tbsp chopped fresh basil
• 1 tsp dried oregano
• Salt and pepper to taste

Instructions:

1. Preheat your oven to 375°F. Lightly grease a baking dish.

2. Using a spoon, scoop out the flesh from the center of each zucchini half, leaving about 1/4 inch of the zucchini shell. Chop the scooped•out zucchini flesh.

3. In a skillet over medium heat, cook the ground turkey, onion, and garlic until the turkey is browned and the vegetables are softened, about 5•7 minutes. Drain any excess fat.

4. Add the chopped zucchini flesh, diced tomatoes, 1/4 cup of the mozzarella cheese, basil, and oregano to the skillet. Season with salt and pepper.

5. Spoon the turkey and vegetable mixture into the hollowed•out zucchini boats, packing it in tightly.

6. Place the stuffed zucchini boats in the prepared baking dish. Top each boat with the remaining 1/4 cup of mozzarella cheese.

7. Bake for 20•25 minutes, until the zucchini is tender and the cheese is melted and bubbly.

8. Serve the stuffed zucchini boats warm.

This stuffed zucchini boat recipe is a delicious and diabetes•friendly meal that combines lean protein, non•starchy vegetables, and healthy fats to help manage blood sugar levels.

23. Tomato and Mozzarella Salad with Basil

Ingredient:

- 1 lb cherry or grape tomatoes, halved
- 8 oz fresh mozzarella cheese, cut into 1•inch cubes
- 1/4 cup fresh basil leaves, chopped
- 2 tbsp olive oil
- 1 tbsp balsamic vinegar
- 1 tsp Dijon mustard
- 1 clove garlic, minced
- Salt and pepper to taste

Instructions:

1. In a large bowl, combine the halved tomatoes, mozzarella cheese cubes, and chopped fresh basil.

2. In a small bowl, whisk together the olive oil, balsamic vinegar, Dijon mustard, and minced garlic. Season with a pinch of salt and pepper.

3. Pour the dressing over the tomato and mozzarella mixture and toss gently to coat.

4. Cover the salad and refrigerate for at least 30 minutes to allow the flavors to meld.

5. Serve the Tomato and Mozzarella Salad chilled or at room temperature.

Tips for a Diabetic Diet:

- Tomatoes are a low•carb, nutrient•dense vegetable that is rich in antioxidants.
- Fresh mozzarella cheese provides protein and healthy fats without significantly increasing carbs.
- Fresh basil adds flavor and antioxidants without any carbs.
- The olive oil and balsamic vinegar dressing is a diabetes•friendly way to add healthy fats and flavor without added sugars.

This Tomato and Mozzarella Salad with Basil is a refreshing and flavorful dish that is well•suited for a diabetic diet. The combination of juicy tomatoes, creamy mozzarella, and fragrant basil, dressed in a simple vinaigrette, makes for a light and satisfying meal or side dish.

The healthy fats, protein, and low•carb ingredients in this salad can help manage blood sugar levels and provide essential nutrients for those with diabetes.

24. Chicken and Vegetable Soup

Ingredient:

• 4 cups low•sodium chicken broth
• 1 lb boneless, skinless chicken breasts, cubed
• 1 cup diced carrots
• 1 cup diced celery
• 1 cup diced onion
• 2 cups chopped kale or spinach
• 1 tsp dried thyme
• 1 tsp dried parsley
• Salt and pepper to taste

Instructions:

1. In a large pot, bring the chicken broth to a simmer over medium heat.

2. Add the cubed chicken, diced carrots, celery, and onion to the pot. Simmer for 10•15 minutes, until the chicken is cooked through and the vegetables are tender.

3. Stir in the chopped kale or spinach and the dried thyme and parsley. Cook for an additional 5 minutes, until the greens are wilted.

4. Season the soup with salt and pepper to taste.

Tips for a Diabetic Diet After 50:

• Chicken is a lean protein that can help stabilize blood sugar levels.
• Carrots, celery, and onions are non•starchy vegetables that provide fiber, vitamins, and minerals without significantly increasing carbs.
• Kale and spinach are nutrient•dense leafy greens that are low in carbs.
• Using low•sodium chicken broth helps control sodium intake, which is important for those with diabetes.
• Herbs and spices like thyme and parsley add flavor without adding sugar or sodium.

This chicken and vegetable soup is a nourishing and diabetes•friendly meal. The combination of lean protein, fiber•rich vegetables, and flavorful herbs and spices makes it an excellent option for those following a diabetic diet after 50.

Serve this soup with a side salad or a small whole grain roll for a complete and balanced meal.

25. Tuna Salad with Greek Yogurt Dressing

Ingredient:

• 2 (5 oz) cans of tuna, drained and flaked
• 1/4 cup plain Greek yogurt
• 1 tbsp Dijon mustard
• 1 tbsp lemon juice
• 1/4 cup diced celery
• 2 tbsp diced red onion
• 2 tbsp chopped parsley
• Salt and pepper to taste
• Lettuce leaves or whole grain crackers, for serving

Instructions:

1. In a medium bowl, combine the flaked tuna, Greek yogurt, Dijon mustard, and lemon juice. Mix well until the dressing is evenly distributed.

2. Fold in the diced celery, red onion, and chopped parsley. Season with salt and pepper to taste.

3. Serve the tuna salad on a bed of lettuce leaves or with whole grain crackers.

Tips for a Diabetic Diet After 50:

• Tuna is an excellent source of lean protein, which can help stabilize blood sugar levels.

• Greek yogurt provides protein and a creamy texture to the dressing, without the added sugars found in mayonnaise•based dressings.

• Dijon mustard and lemon juice add flavor without increasing carbs.

• Celery, onion, and parsley add crunch, flavor, and additional nutrients without significantly raising the carb content.

• Serving the tuna salad on lettuce leaves or with whole grain crackers keeps the carbs low and the fiber high.

This tuna salad with a Greek yogurt dressing is a diabetes•friendly option that is packed with protein, healthy fats, and fiber. It makes for a satisfying and nutritious lunch or snack for those following a diabetic diet after 50.

26. Broccoli and Cheddar Soup

Ingredient:

• 1 tbsp olive oil
• 1 onion, diced
• 2 cloves garlic, minced
• Salt and pepper to taste

• 4 cups low•sodium chicken or vegetable broth
• 4 cups chopped broccoli florets
• 1 cup unsweetened almond milk
• 1/2 cup shredded cheddar cheese
• 1 tbsp cornstarch (optional)

Instructions:

1. In a large pot, heat the olive oil over medium heat. Add the diced onion and sauté for 3•4 minutes until translucent.

2. Add the minced garlic and cook for 1 minute, until fragrant.

3. Pour in the low•sodium broth and add the chopped broccoli florets. Bring the mixture to a simmer and cook for 10•12 minutes, until the broccoli is tender.

4. Carefully transfer the soup to a blender and blend until smooth. Alternatively, use an immersion blender to puree the soup directly in the pot.

5. Return the blended soup to the pot and stir in the unsweetened almond milk.

6. If you'd like a thicker consistency, whisk the cornstarch with a tablespoon of water in a small bowl, then stir it into the soup. Simmer for 2•3 minutes until thickened.

7. Remove the pot from the heat and stir in the shredded cheddar cheese until melted and well combined. Season the soup with salt and pepper to taste.

Tips for a Diabetic Diet After 50:

• Broccoli is a low•carb, high•fiber vegetable that is packed with nutrients.
• Cheddar cheese provides protein and healthy fats without significantly increasing carbs.
• Unsweetened almond milk is a low•carb, dairy•free alternative to regular milk.
• Using low•sodium broth helps control sodium intake, which is important for those with diabetes.
• The cornstarch is optional, as the soup will still be creamy without it.

This broccoli and cheddar soup is a comforting and diabetes•friendly option. The combination of nutrient•dense broccoli, protein•rich cheese, and low•carb almond milk makes it a great choice for those following a diabetic diet after 50.

27. Spinach and Feta Stuffed Chicken Breast

Ingredient:

- 4 boneless, skinless chicken breasts
- 2 cups fresh spinach, chopped
- 1/4 cup crumbled feta cheese
- 1 tbsp olive oil
- 1 clove garlic, minced
- 1/4 tsp dried oregano
- Salt and pepper to taste

Instructions:

1. Preheat your oven to 375°F. Lightly grease a baking dish or line it with parchment paper.

2. In a small bowl, mix together the chopped spinach, crumbled feta, minced garlic, and dried oregano. Season with a pinch of salt and pepper.

3. Using a sharp knife, slice a pocket into the side of each chicken breast, being careful not to cut all the way through.

4. Stuff each chicken breast with about 1/4 of the spinach and feta mixture. Place the stuffed chicken breasts in the prepared baking dish. Drizzle the tops with the olive oil.

5. Bake for 25•30 minutes, until the chicken is cooked through and the internal temperature reaches 165°F. Remove the chicken from the oven and let it rest for 5 minutes before serving.

Tips for a Diabetic Diet After 50:

- Chicken breast is a lean protein that can help stabilize blood sugar levels.
- Spinach is a nutrient•dense leafy green that is low in carbs and high in fiber, vitamins, and minerals.
- Feta cheese provides protein and healthy fats without significantly increasing carbs.
- Olive oil is a source of heart•healthy monounsaturated fats.
- This dish is a complete meal that combines protein, vegetables, and healthy fats to help manage diabetes.

The spinach and feta stuffed chicken breast is a delicious and diabetes•friendly option for those following a diabetic diet after 50. The combination of lean protein, fiber•rich greens, and healthy fats can help regulate blood sugar levels and provide a satisfying meal.

28. Spaghetti Squash with Marinara Sauce

Ingredient:

• 1 medium spaghetti squash, halved lengthwise and seeds removed
• 1 tbsp olive oil
• 1 (24 oz) jar low•sugar marinara sauce
• 1/4 cup grated Parmesan cheese (optional)
• Fresh basil leaves, chopped (optional)
• Salt and pepper to taste

Instructions:

1. Preheat the oven to 400°F. Line a baking sheet with parchment paper.

2. Place the spaghetti squash halves cut•side down on the prepared baking sheet. Roast for 40•50 minutes, until the squash is tender and easily shreds with a fork.

3. Remove the spaghetti squash from the oven and let it cool slightly. Use a fork to shred the flesh of the squash into long, spaghetti•like strands.

4. In a large skillet, heat the olive oil over medium heat. Add the shredded spaghetti squash and sauté for 2•3 minutes to heat through.

5. Pour the low•sugar marinara sauce over the spaghetti squash and toss to coat.

6. Serve the spaghetti squash with marinara sauce, topped with grated Parmesan cheese and fresh chopped basil, if desired.

Tips for a Diabetic Diet After 50:

• Spaghetti squash is a low•carb, high•fiber alternative to traditional pasta, making it a great choice for those with diabetes.
• Low•sugar marinara sauce helps keep the carb and sugar content in check.
• Parmesan cheese provides a boost of protein and healthy fats.
• Fresh basil adds flavor without any additional carbs or sugars.

This spaghetti squash with marinara sauce is a delicious and diabetes•friendly meal. The combination of the low•carb squash, nutrient•dense sauce, and optional toppings makes it a satisfying and blood sugar•friendly option for those following a diabetic diet after 50.

29. Cobb Salad with Turkey Bacon

Ingredient:

- 6 cups chopped romaine lettuce
- 1 cup chopped tomatoes
- 1 avocado, diced
- 1/2 cup cooked turkey bacon, crumbled
- 2 hard boiled eggs, chopped
- 1/4 cup crumbled blue cheese
- 2 tablespoons chopped chives
- 2 tablespoons red wine vinegar
- 1 tablespoon olive oil
- 1 teaspoon Dijon mustard
- Salt and pepper to taste

Instructions:

1. In a large salad bowl, combine the romaine lettuce, tomatoes, avocado, turkey bacon, hard boiled eggs, blue cheese, and chives.

2. In a small bowl, whisk together the red wine vinegar, olive oil, and Dijon mustard. Season with salt and pepper.

3. Drizzle the dressing over the salad and toss gently to coat.

4. Serve immediately.

The combination of crisp romaine, juicy tomatoes, creamy avocado, savory turkey bacon, and tangy blue cheese makes this Cobb salad a delicious and satisfying meal. The homemade vinaigrette ties all the flavors together perfectly. Enjoy!

3O. Black Bean and Corn Salad

Ingredient:

• 1 (15 oz) can black beans, rinsed and drained
• 1 cup frozen corn, thawed
• 1/2 cup diced red onion
• 1/2 cup diced bell pepper (any color)
• 2 tbsp chopped fresh cilantro
• 2 tbsp lime juice
• 1 tbsp olive oil
• 1 tsp ground cumin
• 1/4 tsp chili powder
• Salt and pepper to taste

Instructions:

1. In a large bowl, combine the rinsed and drained black beans, thawed corn, diced red onion, and diced bell pepper.

2. In a small bowl, whisk together the lime juice, olive oil, cumin, and chili powder.

3. Pour the dressing over the bean and vegetable mixture and toss gently to coat.

4. Stir in the chopped fresh cilantro.

5. Season the salad with salt and pepper to taste. Cover and refrigerate for at least 30 minutes to allow the flavors to meld.

Tips for a Diabetic Diet After 50:

• Black beans are a great source of fiber, protein, and complex carbs, which can help regulate blood sugar levels.
• Corn provides fiber and natural sweetness without spiking blood sugar too much.
• Onions, bell peppers, and cilantro add flavor, vitamins, and minerals without significantly increasing carbs.
• The lime juice, olive oil, cumin, and chili powder create a flavorful dressing without added sugars.
• This salad can be served as a side dish or a light main course. It pairs well with grilled chicken or fish.

The black bean and corn salad is a refreshing, diabetes•friendly option that is packed with fiber, protein, and nutrients. It's a great choice for a diabetic diet after 50, providing a balance of complex carbs, healthy fats, and antioxidants.

31. Baked Salmon with Asparagus and Quinoa

Ingredient:

- 4 (6 oz) salmon fillets
- 1 lb asparagus, trimmed
- 1 cup cooked quinoa
- 2 tbsp olive oil
- 2 tbsp lemon juice
- 2 tsp Dijon mustard
- 1 tsp dried dill
- 1/2 tsp garlic powder
- Salt and pepper to taste

Instructions:

1. Preheat oven to 400°F. Line a baking sheet with parchment paper.

2. Place the salmon fillets and asparagus spears on the prepared baking sheet. Drizzle with 1 tbsp of the olive oil and season with salt and pepper.

3. Bake for 12•15 minutes, until the salmon is cooked through and the asparagus is tender.

4. In a small bowl, whisk together the remaining 1 tbsp olive oil, lemon juice, Dijon mustard, dill, and garlic powder. Season with salt and pepper.

5. Divide the cooked quinoa among 4 plates. Top each with a salmon fillet and some of the roasted asparagus.

6. Drizzle the lemon•Dijon dressing over the top.

This dish is perfect for a diabetic diet after 50 as it is high in protein, fiber, and healthy fats from the salmon and quinoa, while being low in carbs. The asparagus provides important vitamins and minerals. The bright lemon•Dijon dressing adds tons of flavor without added sugars. Enjoy this delicious and nutritious meal!

32. Stuffed Bell Peppers with Ground Turkey and Brown Rice

Ingredient:

• 4 large bell peppers, halved lengthwise and seeds/membranes removed
• 1 lb ground turkey
• 1 cup cooked brown rice
• 1 small onion, diced
• 2 cloves garlic, minced
• 1 (14.5 oz) can diced tomatoes
• 2 tbsp tomato paste
• 1 tsp dried oregano
• 1/2 tsp dried basil
• 1/4 tsp red pepper flakes (optional)
• Salt and pepper to taste
• 1/2 cup shredded low•fat mozzarella cheese (optional)

Instructions:

1. Preheat oven to 375°F. Arrange the bell pepper halves in a baking dish.

2. In a large skillet over medium heat, cook the ground turkey, onion, and garlic until the turkey is browned and cooked through, 5•7 minutes. Drain any excess fat.

3. Stir in the cooked brown rice, diced tomatoes, tomato paste, oregano, basil, red pepper flakes (if using), salt, and pepper. Cook for 2•3 minutes.

4. Spoon the turkey•rice mixture evenly into the bell pepper halves.

5. Cover the baking dish with foil and bake for 25•30 minutes, until the peppers are tender.

6. Remove the foil and sprinkle the mozzarella cheese over the tops, if using. Bake for 5 more minutes until the cheese is melted.

7. Serve the stuffed peppers warm.

This dish is perfect for a diabetic diet after 50 as it is high in protein, fiber, and complex carbs from the brown rice and bell peppers, while being low in fat and calories. The ground turkey and cheese are optional, so you can adjust the recipe to your dietary needs. Enjoy this flavorful and healthy stuffed pepper meal!

33. Grilled Shrimp with Zucchini Noodles

Ingredient:

- 1 lb large shrimp, peeled and deveined
- 2 tbsp olive oil
- 1 tsp garlic powder
- 1 tsp paprika
- 1/4 tsp cayenne pepper (optional)
- Salt and pepper to taste
- 3 medium zucchini, spiralized or julienned into noodles
- 2 tbsp lemon juice
- 2 tbsp chopped fresh parsley

Instructions:

1. In a medium bowl, toss the shrimp with 1 tbsp of the olive oil, garlic powder, paprika, cayenne (if using), salt, and pepper.

2. Preheat grill or grill pan to medium·high heat. Thread the shrimp onto skewers.

3. Grill the shrimp for 2·3 minutes per side, until opaque and cooked through. Remove from grill and set aside.

4. In a large skillet, heat the remaining 1 tbsp of olive oil over medium heat. Add the zucchini noodles and sauté for 3·5 minutes, until tender·crisp.

5. Remove the zucchini noodles from heat and toss with the lemon juice and parsley. Season with salt and pepper to taste.

6. Serve the grilled shrimp over the zucchini noodles.

This dish is perfect for a diabetic diet after 50 as it is low in carbs, high in protein and fiber, and features nutrient·dense vegetables. The zucchini noodles provide a healthy alternative to pasta, and the grilled shrimp is a lean source of protein. Enjoy this flavorful and satisfying meal!

34. Roasted Chicken with Brussels Sprouts and Sweet Potatoes

Ingredient:

- 1 lb boneless, skinless chicken breasts
- 1 lb Brussels sprouts, trimmed and halved
- 2 medium sweet potatoes, peeled and cubed
- 2 tbsp olive oil
- 1 tsp dried thyme
- 1 tsp garlic powder
- 1/2 tsp paprika
- Salt and pepper to taste

Instructions:

1. Preheat oven to 400°F. Line a large baking sheet with parchment paper.

2. Place the chicken breasts, Brussels sprouts, and sweet potato cubes on the prepared baking sheet. Drizzle with the olive oil and sprinkle with the thyme, garlic powder, paprika, salt, and pepper. Toss to coat everything evenly.

3. Roast for 25•30 minutes, flipping the vegetables halfway, until the chicken is cooked through (internal temperature reaches 165°F) and the vegetables are tender.

4. Remove from oven and let the chicken rest for 5 minutes before slicing or shredding.

5. Serve the sliced or shredded chicken with the roasted Brussels sprouts and sweet potatoes.

This dish is perfect for a diabetic diet after 50 as it is high in protein, fiber, and complex carbs, while being low in fat and calories. The combination of lean chicken, nutrient•dense vegetables, and complex carbs from the sweet potatoes makes this a well•balanced and satisfying meal. Enjoy!

35. Beef and Broccoli Stir•Fry

Ingredient:

- 1 lb flank steak, thinly sliced against the grain
- 2 tbsp low•sodium soy sauce
- 1 tbsp rice vinegar
- 1 tsp sesame oil
- 1 tsp grated ginger
- 2 cloves garlic, minced
- 1 lb broccoli florets
- 1 tbsp olive oil
- 1/4 cup low•sodium beef broth
- 1 tsp cornstarch
- Salt and pepper to taste
- Chopped green onions for garnish (optional)

Instructions:

1. In a medium bowl, combine the sliced beef, soy sauce, rice vinegar, sesame oil, ginger, and garlic. Toss to coat the beef and let marinate for 15 minutes.

2. In a large skillet or wok, heat the olive oil over high heat. Add the broccoli florets and stir•fry for 2•3 minutes until slightly tender.

3. Add the marinated beef and its marinade to the skillet. Stir•fry for 3•4 minutes until the beef is cooked through.

4. In a small bowl, whisk together the beef broth and cornstarch. Pour this mixture into the skillet and let it simmer for 1•2 minutes until the sauce has thickened.

5. Season with salt and pepper to taste.

6. Serve the beef and broccoli stir•fry over steamed cauliflower rice or zucchini noodles. Garnish with chopped green onions if desired.

This dish is perfect for a diabetic diet after 50 as it is high in protein, low in carbs, and features nutrient•dense broccoli. The simple sauce provides flavor without added sugars. Enjoy this quick and healthy stir•fry!

36. Herb•Crusted Pork Tenderloin with Green Beans

Ingredient:

• 1 lb pork tenderloin
• 2 tbsp chopped fresh rosemary
• 2 tbsp chopped fresh thyme
• 1 tbsp olive oil
• 1 tsp garlic powder
• 1/2 tsp salt
• 1/4 tsp black pepper
• 1 lb green beans, trimmed
• 1 tbsp lemon juice

Instructions:

1. Preheat oven to 400°F. Line a baking sheet with parchment paper.

2. In a small bowl, mix together the rosemary, thyme, olive oil, garlic powder, salt, and pepper.

3. Rub the herb mixture all over the pork tenderloin, coating it evenly.

4. Place the pork tenderloin on the prepared baking sheet. Roast for 20•25 minutes, until the internal temperature reaches 145°F.

5. While the pork is roasting, steam the green beans for 5•7 minutes until tender•crisp. Drain and toss with the lemon juice.

6. Remove the pork from the oven and let it rest for 5 minutes before slicing.

7. Serve the sliced pork tenderloin with the lemon•garlic green beans.

This recipe is perfect for a diabetic diet after 50 as it is high in protein, low in carbs, and features nutrient•dense vegetables. The herb crust adds tons of flavor without adding extra calories or sugar. Enjoy this delicious and healthy pork and green bean dish!

37. Turkey Meatballs with Spaghetti Squash

Ingredient:

- 1 lb ground turkey
- 1/2 cup whole wheat breadcrumbs
- 1/4 cup grated Parmesan cheese
- 1 egg, lightly beaten
- 2 cloves garlic, minced
- 1 tsp dried oregano
- 1/2 tsp salt
- 1/4 tsp black pepper
- 1 medium spaghetti squash, halved and seeded
- 1 (24 oz) jar low•sugar marinara sauce

Instructions:

1. Preheat oven to 400°F. Line a baking sheet with parchment paper.

2. In a large bowl, combine the ground turkey, breadcrumbs, Parmesan, egg, garlic, oregano, salt, and pepper. Mix until well combined.

3. Roll the mixture into 1•inch meatballs and place them on the prepared baking sheet.

4. Bake the meatballs for 18•20 minutes, until cooked through.

5. While the meatballs are baking, place the spaghetti squash halves cut•side down on a baking sheet. Bake for 30•40 minutes, until tender when pierced with a fork.

6. Remove the spaghetti squash from the oven and let cool slightly. Use a fork to shred the squash into spaghetti•like strands.

7. In a large skillet, heat the marinara sauce over medium heat. Add the cooked turkey meatballs and toss to coat.

8. Serve the meatballs and sauce over the spaghetti squash.

This dish is perfect for a diabetic diet after 50 as it is high in protein, low in carbs, and features nutrient•dense vegetables. The spaghetti squash provides a healthy alternative to traditional pasta, and the turkey meatballs are a lean source of protein. Enjoy this flavorful and satisfying meal!

38. Baked Cod with Cauliflower Rice

Ingredient:

- 4 (6 oz) cod fillets
- 2 tbsp olive oil
- 1 tsp paprika
- 1 tsp garlic powder
- 1/2 tsp dried thyme
- 1/4 tsp salt
- 1/4 tsp black pepper
- 4 cups riced cauliflower
- 1 tbsp lemon juice
- 2 tbsp chopped fresh parsley

Instructions:

1. Preheat oven to 400°F. Line a baking sheet with parchment paper.

2. Place the cod fillets on the prepared baking sheet. Drizzle with 1 tbsp of the olive oil and sprinkle with the paprika, garlic powder, thyme, salt, and pepper.

3. Bake for 12•15 minutes, until the cod is opaque and flakes easily with a fork.

4. While the cod is baking, heat the remaining 1 tbsp of olive oil in a large skillet over medium heat. Add the riced cauliflower and sauté for 5•7 minutes, until tender.

5. Remove the cauliflower rice from heat and stir in the lemon juice and chopped parsley. Season with additional salt and pepper to taste.

6. Serve the baked cod fillets over the lemon•parsley cauliflower rice.

This dish is perfect for a diabetic diet after 50 as it is high in protein from the cod, low in carbs from the cauliflower rice, and packed with nutrients. The simple seasoning on the cod keeps it flavorful without added sugars or unhealthy fats. Enjoy this delicious and healthy meal!

39. Vegetarian Chili with Kidney Beans and Lentils

Ingredient:

- 1 tbsp olive oil
- 1 onion, diced
- 3 cloves garlic, minced
- 2 bell peppers, diced
- 2 cups diced tomatoes (canned or fresh)
- 1 (15 oz) can kidney beans, rinsed and drained
- 1 (15 oz) can lentils, rinsed and drained
- 2 tbsp chili powder
- 1 tsp ground cumin
- 1 tsp dried oregano
- 1/2 tsp smoked paprika
- 1/4 tsp cayenne pepper (optional)
- Salt and pepper to taste
- Chopped fresh cilantro for garnish (optional)

Instructions:

1. In a large pot or Dutch oven, heat the olive oil over medium heat. Add the onion and sauté for 5 minutes until translucent.

2. Add the garlic and bell peppers and sauté for 2•3 minutes more.

3. Stir in the diced tomatoes, kidney beans, lentils, chili powder, cumin, oregano, smoked paprika, and cayenne (if using). Season with salt and pepper.

4. Bring the chili to a simmer and let it cook for 20•25 minutes, stirring occasionally, until the flavors have melded and the chili has thickened.

5. Serve the vegetarian chili hot, garnished with chopped fresh cilantro if desired.

This chili is perfect for a diabetic diet after 50 as it is high in fiber, protein, and complex carbs from the beans and lentils, while being low in fat and calories. The blend of spices adds tons of flavor without added sugars. Enjoy this hearty and nutritious vegetarian chili!

4O. Stuffed Portobello Mushrooms with Quinoa and Veggies

Ingredient:

• 4 large portobello mushroom caps, stems removed and chopped
• 1/2 cup cooked quinoa
• 1/2 cup diced bell pepper
• 1/2 cup diced zucchini
• 1/4 cup diced onion
• 2 cloves garlic, minced
• 2 tbsp chopped fresh parsley
• 1 tbsp olive oil
• 1/4 tsp salt
• 1/4 tsp black pepper
• 2 tbsp grated Parmesan cheese (optional)

Instructions:

1. Preheat oven to 400°F. Lightly grease a baking sheet.

2. In a medium skillet, sauté the chopped mushroom stems, bell pepper, zucchini, onion, and garlic in the olive oil over medium heat for 5•7 minutes until vegetables are tender.

3. Remove from heat and stir in the cooked quinoa, parsley, salt, and pepper.

4. Arrange the portobello mushroom caps gill•side up on the prepared baking sheet. Spoon the quinoa mixture evenly into the mushroom caps.

5. Bake for 15•18 minutes, until the mushrooms are tender.

6. Remove from oven and sprinkle the Parmesan cheese over the tops, if using.

7. Serve warm.

This recipe is perfect for a diabetic diet after 50 as it is low in carbs, high in fiber, and packed with nutrient•dense vegetables. The quinoa provides a boost of protein as well. Enjoy this flavorful and healthy stuffed mushroom dish!

41. Lemon Garlic Chicken with Roasted Vegetables

Ingredient:

• 1 lb boneless, skinless chicken breasts
• 2 tbsp olive oil, divided
• 3 cloves garlic, minced
• 2 tbsp lemon juice
• 1 tsp lemon zest
• 1 tsp dried oregano
• 1/2 tsp salt
• 1/4 tsp black pepper
• 1 lb Brussels sprouts, trimmed and halved
• 2 cups cubed butternut squash
• 1 red onion, cut into wedges

Instructions:

1. Preheat oven to 400°F. Line a large baking sheet with parchment paper.

2. In a shallow dish, combine 1 tbsp of the olive oil, garlic, lemon juice, lemon zest, oregano, salt, and pepper. Add the chicken breasts and turn to coat both sides.

3. Arrange the chicken on one side of the prepared baking sheet.

4. In a large bowl, toss the Brussels sprouts, butternut squash, and onion wedges with the remaining 1 tbsp of olive oil. Season with a pinch of salt and pepper.

5. Spread the seasoned vegetables on the other side of the baking sheet, arranging them in a single layer.

6. Roast for 25•30 minutes, flipping the vegetables halfway, until the chicken is cooked through (internal temperature reaches 165°F) and the vegetables are tender.

7. Serve the lemon garlic chicken with the roasted vegetables.

This dish is perfect for a diabetic diet after 50 as it is high in protein, low in carbs, and features a variety of nutrient•dense vegetables. The lemon and garlic flavors add tons of taste without added sugars or unhealthy fats. Enjoy this delicious and healthy meal!

42. Salmon Patties with Mixed Greens

Ingredient:

• 1 (15 oz) can wild•caught salmon, drained and flaked
• 1 egg, lightly beaten
• 2 tbsp whole wheat breadcrumbs
• 2 tbsp finely chopped onion
• 1 tbsp Dijon mustard
• 1 tsp lemon zest
• 1/4 tsp salt
• 1/4 tsp black pepper
• 1 tbsp olive oil
• 5 oz mixed greens
• 1 tbsp olive oil
• 1 tbsp lemon juice
• Salt and pepper to taste

Instructions:

1. In a medium bowl, combine the flaked salmon, egg, breadcrumbs, onion, Dijon mustard, lemon zest, salt, and pepper. Mix well and form into 4 equal•sized patties.

2. In a large skillet, heat 1 tbsp of olive oil over medium heat. Cook the salmon patties for 3•4 minutes per side until golden brown.

3. In a large salad bowl, toss the mixed greens with the remaining 1 tbsp olive oil and lemon juice. Season with salt and pepper.

4. Serve the salmon patties over the dressed mixed greens.

This dish is perfect for a diabetic diet after 50 as it is high in protein from the salmon, low in carbs, and features nutrient•dense greens. The salmon patties are pan•fried instead of deep•fried, keeping the fat and calories in check. Enjoy this delicious and healthy meal!

43. Chicken and Cauliflower Curry

Ingredient:

- 1 lb boneless, skinless chicken breasts, cut into 1•inch pieces
- 1 tbsp olive oil
- 1 onion, diced
- 3 cloves garlic, minced
- 1 tbsp grated fresh ginger
- 2 tsp curry powder
- 1 tsp ground cumin
- 1/2 tsp ground turmeric
- 1/4 tsp cayenne pepper (optional)
- 1 (14 oz) can diced tomatoes
- 1 cup low•sodium chicken broth
- 1 head cauliflower, cut into florets
- 1/4 cup plain Greek yogurt
- 2 tbsp chopped fresh cilantro
- Salt and pepper to taste

Instructions:

1. In a large skillet or Dutch oven, heat the olive oil over medium•high heat. Add the chicken and cook for 3•4 minutes, until lightly browned. Remove the chicken from the pan and set aside.

2. Add the onion to the same pan and sauté for 5 minutes until translucent. Add the garlic, ginger, curry powder, cumin, turmeric, and cayenne (if using). Cook for 1 minute, stirring constantly, until fragrant.

3. Stir in the diced tomatoes and chicken broth. Bring the mixture to a simmer.

4. Add the cauliflower florets to the pan and return the cooked chicken to the curry. Simmer for 15•20 minutes, until the cauliflower is tender and the chicken is cooked through.

5. Remove the curry from heat and stir in the Greek yogurt and chopped cilantro. Season with salt and pepper to taste.

6. Serve the chicken and cauliflower curry over steamed basmati rice or cauliflower rice.

This curry dish is perfect for a diabetic diet after 50 as it is high in protein, low in carbs, and packed with nutrient•dense vegetables. The Greek yogurt adds creaminess without excessive fat or calories. Enjoy this flavorful and healthy curry!

44. Zucchini Lasagna with Ground Beef

Ingredient:

• 2 medium zucchini, sliced lengthwise into 1/4•inch thick strips
• 1 lb lean ground beef
• 1 onion, diced
• 3 cloves garlic, minced
• 1 (28 oz) can crushed tomatoes
• 2 tbsp tomato paste
• 1 tsp dried oregano
• 1/2 tsp dried basil
• 1/4 tsp red pepper flakes (optional)
• Salt and pepper to taste
• 1 cup part•skim ricotta cheese
• 1 egg
• 1/2 cup shredded part•skim mozzarella cheese

Instructions:

1. Preheat oven to 375°F. Grease a 9x13 inch baking dish.

2. In a large skillet over medium heat, cook the ground beef, onion, and garlic until the beef is browned and cooked through, 5•7 minutes. Drain any excess fat.

3. Stir in the crushed tomatoes, tomato paste, oregano, basil, red pepper flakes (if using), and season with salt and pepper. Simmer for 10 minutes.

4. In a small bowl, mix together the ricotta cheese and egg.

5. Arrange a layer of zucchini strips in the bottom of the prepared baking dish. Top with half of the beef•tomato sauce, then dollop half of the ricotta mixture over the sauce. Repeat the layers.

6. Top the lasagna with the shredded mozzarella cheese.

7. Bake for 35•40 minutes, until the cheese is melted and bubbly. Let stand for 5 minutes before serving.

This zucchini lasagna is perfect for a diabetic diet after 50 as it is low in carbs, high in protein, and packed with nutrient•dense vegetables. The lean ground beef and part•skim cheeses keep the fat and calories in check. Enjoy this delicious and healthy twist on traditional lasagna!

45. Eggplant Parmesan with Low•Carb Bread Crumbs

Ingredient:

• 2 medium eggplants, sliced into 1/2•inch thick rounds
• 1/2 cup almond flour
• 1/4 cup grated Parmesan cheese
• 1 tsp dried oregano
• 1/2 tsp garlic powder
• 1/4 tsp salt
• 2 eggs, beaten
• 1 (24 oz) jar low•sugar marinara sauce
• 1 cup shredded part•skim mozzarella cheese

Instructions:

1. Preheat oven to 375°F. Grease a 9x13 inch baking dish.

2. In a shallow bowl, mix together the almond flour, Parmesan cheese, oregano, garlic powder, and salt.

3. Dip the eggplant slices into the beaten eggs, then coat them in the almond flour mixture, pressing to adhere.

4. Arrange the breaded eggplant slices in a single layer in the prepared baking dish.

5. Bake for 20 minutes, flip the eggplant slices, and bake for 15•20 minutes more until golden brown.

6. Spread 1 cup of the marinara sauce in the bottom of the baking dish. Arrange the baked eggplant slices over the sauce.

7. Top the eggplant with the remaining marinara sauce and the shredded mozzarella cheese.

8. Bake for 20•25 minutes, until the cheese is melted and bubbly.

9. Let the eggplant parmesan cool for 5 minutes before serving.

This eggplant parmesan is perfect for a diabetic diet after 50 as it is low in carbs, high in fiber, and features nutrient•dense vegetables. The almond flour and Parmesan coating provides a crispy texture without the need for traditional breadcrumbs. Enjoy this delicious and healthy Italian•inspired dish!

46. Shrimp and Avocado Salad

Ingredient:

• 1 lb cooked shrimp, peeled and deveined
• 2 avocados, diced
• 1 cup cherry tomatoes, halved
• 1/2 red onion, thinly sliced
• 2 tbsp chopped fresh cilantro
• 2 tbsp lime juice
• 1 tbsp olive oil
• 1/4 tsp salt
• 1/4 tsp black pepper
• Mixed greens or baby spinach (optional)

Instructions:

1. In a large bowl, gently toss together the cooked shrimp, diced avocado, cherry tomatoes, red onion, and chopped cilantro.

2. In a small bowl, whisk together the lime juice, olive oil, salt, and pepper to make the dressing.

3. Pour the dressing over the shrimp and avocado mixture and toss gently to coat.

4. Serve the shrimp and avocado salad over a bed of mixed greens or baby spinach, if desired.

This salad is perfect for a diabetic diet after 50 as it is high in protein from the shrimp, healthy fats from the avocado, and fiber from the vegetables. The simple lime•based dressing provides flavor without added sugars. The combination of textures and nutrients makes this a satisfying and nutritious meal.

Enjoy this fresh and flavorful Shrimp and Avocado Salad! It's a great option for a light lunch or dinner.

47. Turkey and Vegetable Skewers

Ingredient:

- 1 lb ground turkey
- 1 zucchini, cut into 1·inch pieces
- 1 red bell pepper, cut into 1·inch pieces
- 1 yellow onion, cut into 1·inch pieces
- 8 oz mushrooms, halved
- 2 tbsp olive oil
- 1 tsp dried oregano
- 1/2 tsp garlic powder
- 1/4 tsp salt
- 1/4 tsp black pepper
- Wooden or metal skewers

Instructions:

1. Preheat grill or grill pan to medium·high heat.

2. In a large bowl, combine the ground turkey, zucchini, bell pepper, onion, and mushrooms. Drizzle with the olive oil and sprinkle with the oregano, garlic powder, salt, and pepper. Toss to coat everything evenly.

3. Thread the turkey and vegetable pieces onto the skewers, alternating the ingredients.

4. Grill the skewers for 12·15 minutes, turning occasionally, until the turkey is cooked through (internal temperature reaches 165°F) and the vegetables are tender.

5. Serve the turkey and vegetable skewers immediately.

This dish is perfect for a diabetic diet after 50 as it is high in protein, low in carbs, and packed with nutrient·dense vegetables. The simple seasoning adds flavor without added sugars or unhealthy fats. Grilling the skewers gives them a delicious smoky char. Enjoy this easy and healthy meal!

You can serve the skewers over a bed of mixed greens or cauliflower rice for a complete and balanced diabetic·friendly dinner.

48. Cabbage Rolls with Ground Chicken

Ingredient:

- 1 medium head green cabbage
- 1 lb ground chicken
- 1/2 cup cooked brown rice
- 1 egg, lightly beaten
- 1/4 cup grated Parmesan cheese
- 2 cloves garlic, minced
- 1 tsp dried oregano
- 1/2 tsp salt
- 1/4 tsp black pepper
- 1 (15 oz) can tomato sauce
- 1/4 cup low•sodium chicken broth

Instructions:

1. Bring a large pot of water to a boil. Add the whole head of cabbage and cook for 3•5 minutes until the outer leaves are softened. Remove the cabbage and let cool slightly.

2. Carefully peel off the softened cabbage leaves, keeping them intact. You should have about 12•14 leaves.

3. In a medium bowl, combine the ground chicken, cooked brown rice, egg, Parmesan, garlic, oregano, salt, and pepper. Mix well.

4. Place about 2•3 tablespoons of the chicken mixture onto the center of each cabbage leaf. Fold the sides of the leaf over the filling, then roll up tightly.

5. Arrange the stuffed cabbage rolls seam•side down in a 9x13 inch baking dish.

6. In a small bowl, whisk together the tomato sauce and chicken broth. Pour this sauce over the cabbage rolls.

7. Cover the baking dish with foil and bake at 375°F for 45•55 minutes, until the cabbage is tender and the filling is cooked through.

8. Serve the cabbage rolls warm, with the sauce spooned over the top.

This dish is perfect for a diabetic diet after 50 as it is high in protein, low in carbs, and features nutrient•dense cabbage. The ground chicken and brown rice filling provides a satisfying and healthy meal. Enjoy these delicious and easy cabbage rolls!

49. Chicken Stir•Fry with Snow Peas and Bell Peppers

Ingredient:

- 1 lb boneless, skinless chicken breasts, cut into 1•inch pieces
- 2 tbsp low•sodium soy sauce
- 1 tbsp rice vinegar
- 1 tsp sesame oil
- 1 tsp grated ginger
- 2 cloves garlic, minced
- 1 tbsp olive oil
- 1 red bell pepper, sliced
- 1 yellow bell pepper, sliced
- 8 oz snow peas, trimmed
- 2 green onions, sliced
- 1/4 cup low•sodium chicken broth
- 1 tsp cornstarch
- Salt and pepper to taste
- Cooked brown rice, for serving (optional)

Instructions:

1. In a medium bowl, combine the chicken, soy sauce, rice vinegar, sesame oil, ginger, and garlic. Toss to coat the chicken and let marinate for 15 minutes.

2. Heat the olive oil in a large skillet or wok over high heat. Add the marinated chicken and stir•fry for 3•4 minutes until lightly browned.

3. Add the bell pepper slices and snow peas to the skillet. Stir•fry for 2•3 minutes until the vegetables are crisp•tender.

4. In a small bowl, whisk together the chicken broth and cornstarch. Pour this mixture into the skillet and let it simmer for 1•2 minutes until the sauce has thickened.

5. Remove from heat and stir in the sliced green onions. Season with salt and pepper to taste.

6. Serve the chicken stir•fry over cooked brown rice, if desired.

This dish is perfect for a diabetic diet after 50 as it is high in protein, low in carbs, and packed with nutrient•dense vegetables. The simple sauce provides flavor without added sugars. Enjoy this quick and healthy stir•fry!

50. Baked Tilapia with Spinach and Tomatoes

Ingredient:

• 4 (6 oz) tilapia fillets
• 2 tbsp olive oil
• 2 cloves garlic, minced
• 1 (14.5 oz) can diced tomatoes, drained
• 4 cups fresh spinach
• 1/4 cup low•sodium chicken or vegetable broth
• 1 tsp dried oregano
• 1/4 tsp salt
• 1/4 tsp black pepper

Instructions:

1. Preheat oven to 400°F. Lightly grease a 9x13 inch baking dish.

2. Place the tilapia fillets in the prepared baking dish. Drizzle with 1 tbsp of the olive oil and season with salt and pepper.

3. In a large skillet, heat the remaining 1 tbsp of olive oil over medium heat. Add the garlic and sauté for 1 minute until fragrant.

4. Add the drained diced tomatoes, spinach, broth, oregano, salt, and pepper. Cook for 2•3 minutes, stirring occasionally, until the spinach is wilted.

5. Spoon the spinach and tomato mixture over the top of the tilapia fillets.

6. Bake for 15•18 minutes, until the fish flakes easily with a fork and is cooked through.

7. Serve the baked tilapia immediately, with the spinach and tomatoes spooned over the top.

This dish is perfect for a diabetic diet after 50 as it is high in protein, low in carbs, and packed with nutrient•dense vegetables. The tilapia is a lean, mild•flavored fish that pairs beautifully with the garlicky spinach and tomatoes. Enjoy this delicious and healthy baked fish meal!

51. Apple Slices with Almond Butter

Ingredient:

• 1 medium apple, cored and sliced
• 2 tbsp natural almond butter

Instructions:

1. Wash and slice the apple into thin wedges or rounds.

2. Scoop the almond butter into a small serving dish or bowl.

3. Arrange the apple slices around the almond butter, using them as "dippers" to enjoy the nut butter.

That's it! This simple snack is a great option for those following a diabetic diet after 50.

The benefits of this dish include:

• Apples are a good source of fiber and provide natural sweetness without a lot of sugar.
• Almond butter is high in healthy fats, protein, and fiber, which can help keep blood sugar levels stable.
• This combination provides a satisfying and nutritious snack that is low in carbs and calories.

You can use any variety of apple you prefer, such as Gala, Fuji, or Honeycrisp. Just be mindful of portion sizes, as even though apples are a healthy fruit, they do contain natural sugars.

Enjoy this simple and delicious snack of apple slices with almond butter as part of a diabetic•friendly diet after 50. It's a great way to satisfy cravings for something sweet and creamy while supporting your overall health.

52. Cucumber Slices with Hummus

Ingredient:

• 1 medium cucumber, sliced into rounds or spears
• 1/2 cup plain, unsweetened Greek yogurt•based hummus

Instructions:

1. Wash and slice the cucumber into rounds or spears, depending on your preference.

2. Scoop the hummus into a small serving bowl or dish.

3. Arrange the cucumber slices around the hummus, using them as "dippers" to enjoy the hummus.

That's it! This simple snack is a great option for those following a diabetic diet after 50.

The benefits of this dish include:

• Cucumbers are low in carbs, high in water content, and provide a crunchy, refreshing texture.
• Hummus is made from chickpeas, which are a good source of fiber and protein. The Greek yogurt•based hummus also adds a boost of protein.
• This combination provides a satisfying snack that is low in calories and carbs, while still being flavorful and filling.

You can use any variety of hummus you enjoy, such as classic, roasted red pepper, or even a lower•fat or reduced•sodium version to further customize it for your dietary needs.

Enjoy this simple and healthy snack of cucumber slices with hummus as a diabetic•friendly option after 50. It's a great way to curb hunger and satisfy cravings in a nutritious way.

53. Mixed Nuts

Ingredient:

• 1/4 cup mixed nuts (such as almonds, walnuts, pecans, cashews, etc.)

Instructions:

1. Measure out a 1/4 cup serving of your desired mixed nuts.

That's it! This simple snack of mixed nuts is a great option for those following a diabetic diet after 50.

The benefits of mixed nuts include:

• Nuts are high in healthy fats, protein, and fiber, which can help keep blood sugar levels stable.
• They provide a satisfying crunch and flavor that can help curb hunger and cravings.
• Nuts contain important vitamins, minerals, and antioxidants that support overall health.

When choosing a mix of nuts, try to select a variety that is unsalted and unsweetened. Avoid nuts that are coated in sugar, honey, or other sweeteners.

A 1/4 cup serving of mixed nuts is a good portion size to aim for as part of a diabetic diet. The healthy fats and protein will help you feel full and satisfied without spiking your blood sugar.

Enjoy this simple, nutrient•dense snack of mixed nuts as a diabetic•friendly option after 50. It's a great way to get a boost of energy and nutrition between meals.

54. Greek Yogurt with a Dash of Cinnamon

Ingredient:

• 1 cup plain, unsweetened Greek yogurt
• 1/4 tsp ground cinnamon

Instructions:

1. Scoop the Greek yogurt into a serving bowl or dish.

2. Sprinkle the ground cinnamon evenly over the top of the yogurt.

That's it! This easy snack or light breakfast is a great option for those following a diabetic diet after 50.

The benefits of this dish include:

• Greek yogurt is high in protein and low in carbs, making it an excellent choice for diabetics. The protein helps keep you feeling full and satisfied.

• Cinnamon is a spice that may help regulate blood sugar levels. It also adds a warm, sweet flavor without any added sugar.

• This simple combination provides a nutritious and delicious treat that is quick and easy to prepare.

You can enjoy this Greek yogurt with cinnamon on its own, or you can top it with a small amount of fresh berries, chopped nuts, or a drizzle of honey if desired. Just be mindful of portion sizes and additional toppings to keep the carb and calorie counts in check.

This healthy snack is a great way to satisfy your sweet tooth while supporting your diabetic diet after 50. Enjoy!

55. Carrot Sticks with Guacamole

Ingredient:

• 2•3 medium carrots, peeled and cut into sticks
• 1/2 cup homemade or store•bought guacamole

Instructions:

1. Wash, peel, and cut the carrots into 3•4 inch sticks.

2. Scoop the guacamole into a small serving bowl or dish.

3. Arrange the carrot sticks around the guacamole, using them as "dippers" to enjoy the creamy avocado dip.

That's it! This simple snack is a great option for those following a diabetic diet after 50.

The benefits of this dish include:

• Carrots are a low•carb, high•fiber vegetable that is rich in vitamins and minerals.
• Guacamole is made from avocados, which provide healthy fats and fiber to help stabilize blood sugar levels.
• This combination offers a satisfying and nutrient•dense snack that is easy to prepare.

You can make your own guacamole at home using ripe avocados, lime juice, onion, cilantro, and seasonings. Or you can use a store•bought version that is low in added sugars and oils.

Be mindful of portion sizes, as even healthy fats from avocados can be high in calories. Stick to a 1/2 cup serving of guacamole.

Enjoy this simple and delicious snack of carrot sticks with guacamole as part of a diabetic•friendly diet after 50. It's a great way to get in some extra vegetables and healthy fats.

56. Celery Sticks with Peanut Butter

Ingredient:

• 2•3 stalks of celery, cut into 3•4 inch sticks
• 2 tbsp natural, unsweetened peanut butter

Instructions:

1. Wash and cut the celery stalks into 3•4 inch sticks.

2. Scoop the peanut butter into a small serving dish or bowl.

3. Arrange the celery sticks around the peanut butter, using them as "dippers" to enjoy the nut butter.

That's it! This simple snack is a great option for those following a diabetic diet after 50.

The benefits of this dish include:

• Celery is very low in carbs and calories, making it a great vegetable choice for diabetics.
• Peanut butter is high in healthy fats and protein, which can help stabilize blood sugar levels.
• This combination provides a satisfying and nutritious snack that is easy to prepare.

You can use any type of natural, unsweetened peanut butter for this recipe. Avoid peanut butters with added sugars or oils.

Be mindful of portion sizes, as even healthy nut butters can be high in calories. Stick to a 2 tbsp serving of peanut butter.

Enjoy this simple and delicious snack of celery sticks with peanut butter as part of a diabetic•friendly diet after 50. It's a great way to curb hunger and satisfy cravings in a nutritious way.

57. Hard•Boiled Eggs

Ingredient:

• 2•3 large eggs

Instructions:

1. Place the eggs in a single layer in a saucepan and cover with cold water by 1 inch.

2. Bring the water to a boil over high heat. Once the water reaches a full boil, remove the pan from the heat and cover.

3. Let the eggs sit in the hot water for 12 minutes for large eggs. Adjust the time up or down by a minute or two for smaller or larger eggs.

4. Drain the hot water and cover the eggs with cold water to stop the cooking. Let sit for 5 minutes.

5. Peel the eggs and enjoy!

Hard•boiled eggs are an excellent snack or addition to meals for those following a diabetic diet after 50. Here's why:

• Eggs are high in protein, which helps keep you feeling full and satisfied.
• They contain no carbs, making them a great low•carb option.
• Eggs are packed with important vitamins and minerals like vitamin B12, selenium, and choline.
• They are easy to prepare in advance and take on the go as a portable, nutrient•dense snack.

You can enjoy hard•boiled eggs on their own, or pair them with other diabetic•friendly foods like sliced avocado, a small amount of hummus, or a sprinkle of salt and pepper.

Hard•boiled eggs are a simple, versatile, and nutritious option to incorporate into your diabetic diet after 50. Give this easy recipe a try!

58. Cheese and Whole Grain Crackers

Ingredient:

• 1•2 oz low•fat or reduced•fat cheese, sliced or cubed
• 6•8 whole grain crackers

Instructions:

1. Choose a low•fat or reduced•fat cheese, such as cheddar, Swiss, or mozzarella.

2. Slice or cube the cheese into bite•sized pieces.

3. Arrange the cheese cubes or slices on a plate alongside the whole grain crackers.

This simple snack of cheese and whole grain crackers is a great option for those following a diabetic diet after 50.

The benefits of this combination include:

• Cheese provides protein and healthy fats to help keep you feeling full and satisfied.
• Whole grain crackers offer complex carbohydrates, fiber, and important nutrients.
• The combination of protein, fat, and fiber helps to stabilize blood sugar levels.

When selecting the cheese and crackers, look for options that are low in added sugars and sodium. Opt for reduced•fat or low•fat cheeses, and choose whole grain crackers that are high in fiber and low in carbs.

A serving size of 1•2 oz of cheese and 6•8 crackers is a good portion to aim for as part of a diabetic diet after 50. This provides a balanced snack that is satisfying and nutritious.

Enjoy this simple and easy•to•prepare snack of cheese and whole grain crackers as a diabetic•friendly option. It's a great way to curb hunger and provide your body with important nutrients.

59. Berries with Cottage Cheese

Ingredient:

- 1 cup low•fat or non•fat cottage cheese
- 1 cup mixed berries (such as blueberries, raspberries, and/or blackberries)
- 1 tsp honey (optional)
- 1 tbsp chopped walnuts or sliced almonds (optional)

Instructions:

1. Scoop the cottage cheese into a serving bowl or dish.

2. Top the cottage cheese with the mixed berries.

3. If desired, drizzle the honey over the top of the berries and cottage cheese.

4. Sprinkle the chopped walnuts or sliced almonds over the top, if using.

That's it! This simple and delicious snack or light meal is perfect for a diabetic diet after 50.

The benefits of this dish include:

- Cottage cheese is high in protein and low in carbs, making it a great choice for diabetics.

- Berries are packed with antioxidants, fiber, and natural sweetness without a lot of sugar.

- Nuts provide healthy fats and additional fiber.

- The optional honey adds a touch of sweetness if desired, but can be omitted.

This combination of protein, fiber, and healthy fats will help keep blood sugar levels stable. Enjoy this refreshing and nutritious treat!

60. Olives and Cherry Tomatoes

Ingredient:

• 1/4 cup mixed olives (such as Kalamata, green, or black)
• 1/2 cup cherry or grape tomatoes, halved

Instructions:

1. Rinse and drain the olives.

2. Wash the cherry or grape tomatoes and slice them in half.

3. Arrange the olives and tomato halves on a small plate or in a bowl.

This simple snack of olives and cherry tomatoes is a great option for those following a diabetic diet after 50.

The benefits of this combination include:

• Olives are a good source of healthy monounsaturated fats, which can help regulate blood sugar levels.
• Cherry tomatoes are low in carbs and high in vitamins, minerals, and antioxidants.
• The combination provides a flavorful, crunchy, and nutrient•dense snack.

When selecting the olives, choose ones that are packed in water or brine, rather than oil. Avoid olives with added sugars or sodium.

A serving size of 1/4 cup olives and 1/2 cup cherry tomatoes is a good portion to aim for as part of a diabetic diet after 50. This provides a balanced snack that is satisfying and nutritious.

Enjoy this simple and easy•to•prepare snack of olives and cherry tomatoes as a diabetic•friendly option. It's a great way to curb hunger and provide your body with important nutrients.

61. Edamame with Sea Salt

Ingredient:

• 1 lb frozen edamame in the pod
• 1 tsp sea salt

Instructions:

1. Bring a large pot of water to a boil over high heat.

2. Add the frozen edamame pods to the boiling water. Cook for 5•7 minutes, until the pods are bright green and tender.

3. Drain the edamame and transfer to a serving bowl.

4. Sprinkle the sea salt over the hot edamame and toss to coat evenly.

5. Serve the edamame warm, with the pods intact. Provide a small bowl for discarding the empty pods.

Nutritional Info (per 1/2 cup serving):
• Calories: 100
• Total Carbs: 9g
• Fiber: 4g
• Net Carbs: 5g
• Protein: 9g
• Fat: 4.5g

Edamame is an excellent source of plant•based protein, fiber, and micronutrients like folate and vitamin K. The sea salt adds flavor without adding sugar or excessive sodium. This makes a great diabetic•friendly snack or appetizer.

Edamame is low in calories and carbs, and the fiber and protein help keep blood sugar levels stable. It's a healthy, satisfying option for those following a diabetic diet after 50.

62. Pumpkin Seeds

Ingredient:

• 1 cup raw pumpkin seeds (pepitas)
• 1 tsp olive oil
• 1/2 tsp ground cumin
• 1/4 tsp garlic powder
• 1/4 tsp salt
• 1/8 tsp cayenne pepper (optional, for a little kick)

Instructions:

1. Preheat your oven to 325°F. Line a baking sheet with parchment paper.

2. In a small bowl, toss the pumpkin seeds with the olive oil, cumin, garlic powder, salt, and cayenne (if using) until the seeds are evenly coated.

3. Spread the seasoned pumpkin seeds in a single layer on the prepared baking sheet.

4. Roast for 12•15 minutes, stirring halfway, until the seeds are lightly golden brown and fragrant.

5. Allow the roasted pumpkin seeds to cool completely before serving.

Nutritional Info (per 1/4 cup serving):
• Calories: 90
• Total Carbs: 3g
• Fiber: 2g
• Net Carbs: 1g
• Protein: 5g
• Fat: 7g

Pumpkin seeds are an excellent source of magnesium, zinc, and healthy fats. The roasting process brings out their nutty, savory flavor. These make a great diabetic•friendly snack or topping for salads, yogurt, or oatmeal. Enjoy in moderation as part of a balanced diet.

63. Bell Pepper Strips with Tzatziki

Ingredient:

For the Tzatziki Dip:
• 1 cup plain Greek yogurt
• 1/2 cucumber, peeled, seeded and finely chopped
• 1 tbsp fresh lemon juice
• 1 tsp minced garlic
• 1/4 tsp salt
• 1/4 tsp black pepper

For the Bell Pepper Strips:
• 2 large bell peppers (any color), washed and sliced into long, thin strips

Instructions:

1. Make the tzatziki dip: In a medium bowl, combine the Greek yogurt, chopped cucumber, lemon juice, garlic, salt and pepper. Stir well to mix. Cover and refrigerate until ready to serve.

2. Prepare the bell pepper strips: Wash the bell peppers and slice them into long, thin strips, about 1/2•inch wide.

3. Arrange the bell pepper strips on a serving platter.

4. Serve the chilled tzatziki dip alongside the bell pepper strips for dipping.

Nutritional Info (per 1/4 cup tzatziki + 1/2 cup bell pepper strips):
• Calories: 60
• Total Carbs: 7g
• Fiber: 2g
• Net Carbs: 5g
• Protein: 5g
• Fat: 1.5g

This makes a refreshing, crunchy and nutrient•dense snack or appetizer for diabetics. The bell peppers provide fiber, vitamins and antioxidants, while the tzatziki dip is high in protein and low in carbs. It's a great way to enjoy a satisfying, diabetes•friendly treat.

64. Roasted Chickpeas

Ingredient:

• 1 (15 oz) can chickpeas (garbanzo beans), drained and rinsed
• 1 tbsp olive oil
• 1 tsp paprika
• 1/2 tsp garlic powder
• 1/4 tsp salt
• 1/4 tsp black pepper

Instructions:

1. Preheat oven to 400°F. Line a baking sheet with parchment paper.

2. Pat the chickpeas dry with a paper towel to remove any excess moisture.

3. In a bowl, toss the chickpeas with the olive oil, paprika, garlic powder, salt, and pepper until evenly coated.

4. Spread the chickpeas in a single layer on the prepared baking sheet.

5. Roast for 20•25 minutes, stirring halfway, until the chickpeas are crispy.

6. Allow to cool slightly before serving.

Nutritional Info (per serving, about 1/4 cup):
• Calories: 120
• Total Carbs: 16g
• Fiber: 5g
• Net Carbs: 11g
• Protein: 6g
• Fat: 4g

These roasted chickpeas make a great high•fiber, high•protein snack for diabetics. The spices add flavor without added sugar. Enjoy them as a crunchy topping on salads or as a standalone snack.

65. Dark Chocolate Squares (in moderation)

Ingredient:

• 1 oz (1•2 squares) of high•quality dark chocolate (70% cacao or higher)

Instructions:

1. Choose a small portion of dark chocolate, around 1•2 squares (1 oz).

2. Savor the dark chocolate slowly, taking the time to appreciate the rich, complex flavors.

Nutritional Info (per 1 oz serving):
• Calories: 170
• Total Carbs: 12g
• Fiber: 3g
• Net Carbs: 9g
• Protein: 2g
• Fat: 12g

Dark chocolate can be a great treat for diabetics when consumed in moderation. Here's why it can be a good option:

• High in Antioxidants: Dark chocolate is rich in flavanols, which are powerful antioxidants that may help reduce inflammation.

• Moderate Carb Content: Compared to milk chocolate, dark chocolate has a lower carb and sugar content, making it a better choice for diabetics.

• Satisfying Flavor: The intense, complex flavor of dark chocolate can be very satisfying in small portions, curbing cravings for sweets.

The key is to stick to a small, controlled portion of 1•2 squares (1 oz) of high•quality dark chocolate with 70% cacao or higher. This provides just enough sweetness and richness without spiking blood sugar too much.

Enjoy the dark chocolate slowly and mindfully as an occasional treat. Pair it with a cup of herbal tea or a handful of nuts for a more balanced snack. As with any food, moderation is key for diabetics.

66. Turkey Roll•Ups with Cheese

Ingredient:

• 4 oz thinly sliced turkey breast
• 1 oz low•fat cheddar or Swiss cheese, sliced
• 1 tbsp cream cheese, softened
• 1 tsp Dijon mustard
• 1/4 tsp dried herbs (such as oregano or basil)
• Salt and pepper to taste

Instructions:

1. In a small bowl, mix together the cream cheese, Dijon mustard, and dried herbs until well combined.

2. Lay the turkey slices out flat on a clean surface. Spread a thin layer of the cream cheese mixture evenly over each slice.

3. Place a slice of cheese on the edge of each turkey slice. Carefully roll up the turkey around the cheese, securing with a toothpick if needed.

4. Arrange the turkey roll•ups on a plate or platter. Refrigerate until ready to serve.

Nutritional Info (per 2 roll•up serving):
• Calories: 120
• Total Carbs: 2g
• Fiber: 0g
• Net Carbs: 2g
• Protein: 15g
• Fat: 6g

These turkey roll•ups make a great diabetic•friendly snack or light meal. The combination of lean protein from the turkey, healthy fats from the cheese, and minimal carbs helps keep blood sugar levels stable.

The cream cheese and mustard add flavor without added sugars. You can customize the herbs and cheese to your taste preferences. Serve these roll•ups with a side of fresh veggies for a complete, diabetes•friendly meal.

67. Kale Chips

Ingredient:

• 1 bunch kale, washed and dried thoroughly
• 1 tbsp olive oil
• 1/4 tsp salt
• 1/4 tsp black pepper

Instructions:

1. Preheat your oven to 325°F. Line a large baking sheet with parchment paper.

2. Tear the kale leaves off the tough stems and into bite•sized pieces. Place the kale in a large bowl.

3. Drizzle the kale with the olive oil and sprinkle with the salt and pepper. Toss gently to coat the kale evenly.

4. Spread the kale pieces in a single layer on the prepared baking sheet, making sure they don't overlap.

5. Bake for 12•15 minutes, flipping the kale halfway, until the leaves are crispy and lightly browned.

6. Remove the kale chips from the oven and let cool completely before serving.

Nutritional Info (per 1 cup serving):
• Calories: 50
• Total Carbs: 6g
• Fiber: 2g
• Net Carbs: 4g
• Protein: 2g
• Fat: 3g

Kale chips make a fantastic diabetic•friendly snack. Kale is low in carbs, high in fiber, and packed with vitamins, minerals and antioxidants. The baking process transforms the leaves into a crispy, satisfying chip•like texture.

These kale chips are seasoned simply with just olive oil, salt and pepper, keeping the carb and calorie counts low. They're a great alternative to traditional potato chips or other high•carb snacks. Enjoy them as a crunchy, nutrient•dense treat!

68. Low•Sugar Protein Bar

Ingredient:

• Protein Blend (Milk Protein Isolate, Soluble Corn Fiber, Erythritol, Almonds, Peanuts)
• Soluble Corn Fiber
• Erythritol
• Cocoa Butter
• Peanut Flour
• Almonds
• Unsweetened Chocolate
• Chicory Root Fiber
• Sea Salt
• Stevia Leaf Extract
• Natural Flavors

Nutritional Info (per bar):
• Calories: 190
• Total Carbs: 21g
• Fiber: 15g
• Net Carbs: 6g
• Protein: 20g
• Fat: 9g

The Quest Nutrition Protein Bar is an excellent option for diabetics looking for a low•sugar, high•protein snack. Here's why it's a good choice:

• Low in Net Carbs: With only 6g of net carbs per bar, it won't spike blood sugar levels.

• High in Fiber: The 15g of fiber helps slow the absorption of carbs.

• Sweetened with Erythritol: A zero•calorie, non•glycemic sweetener that doesn't affect blood sugar.

• Good Source of Protein: 20g of protein per bar helps promote satiety and stable energy.

• Minimal Added Sugars: No high fructose corn syrup or other added sugars.

These protein bars can be a convenient, diabetes•friendly snack or mini•meal. They provide a balance of protein, fiber, and healthy fats to help manage blood sugar. Just be mindful of portion sizes, as even low•sugar bars should be consumed in moderation as part of an overall healthy diet.

69. Almonds and Dried Apricots

Ingredient:

• 1/4 cup raw, unsalted almonds
• 2 tablespoons dried, unsweetened apricots, chopped

Instructions:

1. Combine the almonds and chopped dried apricots in a small bowl or resealable bag.

Nutritional Information (per serving):
• Calories: 150
• Total Carbs: 12g
• Fiber: 4g
• Net Carbs: 8g
• Protein: 5g
• Fat: 10g

This simple snack provides a nice balance of healthy fats, fiber, and natural sweetness for diabetics. Here's why it's a great choice:

Almonds:
• High in healthy monounsaturated fats, protein, and fiber to help manage blood sugar.
• Contain magnesium, which is important for insulin sensitivity.

Dried Apricots:
• Provide natural sweetness from fruit sugars.
• High in fiber to slow the absorption of sugars.
• Rich in vitamins and antioxidants.

The combination of the crunchy almonds and chewy apricots makes for a satisfying, nutrient•dense snack. The portion size of 1/4 cup almonds and 2 tbsp apricots keeps the carbs and calories in check for a diabetic diet.

This makes an easy, portable snack that can help curb hunger and stabilize blood sugar levels. Enjoy it as a midday pick•me•up or as part of a balanced diabetic•friendly meal plan.

70. Mini Caprese Salad Skewers

Ingredient:

- 12 cherry tomatoes, halved
- 12 small fresh mozzarella balls (bocconcini)
- 12 fresh basil leaves
- 2 tbsp balsamic glaze
- 1 tsp extra virgin olive oil
- 1/4 tsp salt
- 1/8 tsp black pepper

Instructions:

1. Assemble the skewers by threading a tomato half, a mozzarella ball, and a basil leaf onto each toothpick or small skewer.

2. Arrange the caprese skewers on a serving platter.

3. In a small bowl, whisk together the balsamic glaze and olive oil. Drizzle this dressing over the caprese skewers.

4. Sprinkle the skewers with salt and pepper.

5. Serve immediately or refrigerate until ready to serve.

Nutritional Info (per 2 skewer serving):
- Calories: 80
- Total Carbs: 4g
- Fiber: 1g
- Net Carbs: 3g
- Protein: 5g
- Fat: 5g

These mini caprese salad skewers are a perfect diabetic•friendly appetizer or snack. The combination of juicy tomatoes, creamy mozzarella, and fresh basil provides a burst of flavor.

The balsamic glaze dressing adds a touch of sweetness without spiking blood sugar levels. The portion size of 2 skewers keeps the carb and calorie counts in check.

Caprese salad is naturally low in carbs and high in healthy fats and protein, making it an excellent choice for diabetics. These easy•to•assemble skewers are a visually appealing and tasty way to enjoy this classic Italian salad.

71. Zucchini Bread with Almond Flour

Ingredient:

• 2 cups grated zucchini (about 1 medium zucchini)
• 1 1/2 cups almond flour
• 1/4 cup granulated erythritol or monk fruit sweetener
• 2 large eggs
• 1/4 cup unsweetened applesauce
• 1 tsp baking powder
• 1 tsp ground cinnamon
• 1/4 tsp salt

Instructions:

1. Preheat your oven to 350°F. Grease a 9x5 inch loaf pan with non•stick cooking spray.

2. Grate the zucchini using a box grater or food processor. Squeeze out any excess moisture from the grated zucchini.

3. In a large bowl, whisk together the almond flour, erythritol/monk fruit, eggs, applesauce, baking powder, cinnamon and salt until well combined.

4. Fold in the grated zucchini until evenly distributed.

5. Pour the batter into the prepared loaf pan and smooth the top.

6. Bake for 45•55 minutes, until a toothpick inserted in the center comes out clean.

7. Allow the zucchini bread to cool in the pan for 10 minutes, then transfer to a wire rack to cool completely before slicing.

This zucchini bread is a great option for diabetics as it's made with low•carb almond flour instead of traditional wheat flour. The grated zucchini adds moisture and nutrients without significantly increasing the carb content. The natural sweetness from the applesauce and cinnamon means you can use less added sweetener.

Enjoy a slice of this moist, flavorful zucchini bread as a snack or light breakfast. It's a diabetes•friendly baked good that can satisfy your sweet tooth.

72. Greek Yogurt Parfait with Nuts and Berries

Ingredient:

• 1 cup plain, unsweetened Greek yogurt
• 1/2 cup fresh berries (such as blueberries, raspberries, or blackberries)
• 2 tbsp chopped walnuts or almonds
• 1 tsp honey or maple syrup (optional)

Instructions:

1. In a parfait glass or bowl, layer half of the Greek yogurt.

2. Top the yogurt with half of the fresh berries and half of the chopped nuts.

3. Repeat the layers, ending with the remaining yogurt, berries, and nuts.

4. If desired, drizzle the top with a small amount of honey or maple syrup.

5. Serve chilled.

Nutritional Info (per parfait):
• Calories: 200
• Total Carbs: 15g
• Fiber: 4g
• Net Carbs: 11g
• Protein: 15g
• Fat: 10g

This Greek yogurt parfait is an excellent diabetic•friendly snack or light meal. Here's why it's a great choice:

• Greek yogurt is high in protein to help stabilize blood sugar.
• Berries are low in carbs and high in fiber, vitamins, and antioxidants.
• Nuts provide healthy fats and a crunchy texture.
• The optional honey or maple syrup adds just a touch of natural sweetness.

The combination of protein, fiber, and healthy fats helps slow the absorption of carbs, preventing blood sugar spikes. This parfait is also very satisfying and can help curb hunger.

Feel free to adjust the portions or swap in different berries and nuts to suit your taste preferences. This makes a refreshing, nutrient•dense treat that fits well into a diabetic diet.

73. Sweet Potato and Black Bean Breakfast Burrito

Ingredient:

• 1 medium sweet potato, peeled and diced
• 1 (15 oz) can black beans, rinsed and drained
• 4 large eggs, scrambled
• 2 tbsp salsa
• 1 tbsp chopped fresh cilantro
• 1/4 tsp ground cumin
• 1/4 tsp chili powder
• 2 whole wheat tortillas (8•inch size)

Instructions:

1. In a skillet over medium heat, sauté the diced sweet potato until tender, about 8•10 minutes.

2. Add the black beans, scrambled eggs, salsa, cilantro, cumin, and chili powder. Stir to combine and heat through.

3. Warm the tortillas according to package instructions.

4. Divide the sweet potato•black bean•egg mixture evenly between the two tortillas.

5. Fold the bottom of each tortilla up, then fold in the sides and roll up tightly to create a burrito. Serve the breakfast burritos warm.

Nutritional Info (per burrito):
• Calories: 350
• Total Carbs: 45g
• Fiber: 9g
• Net Carbs: 36g
• Protein: 17g
• Fat: 10g

This sweet potato and black bean breakfast burrito is a great diabetic•friendly option. The combination of high•fiber sweet potatoes, protein•rich eggs, and nutrient•dense black beans helps keep blood sugar levels stable. The salsa, cilantro, cumin, and chili powder add flavor without added sugars. Whole wheat tortillas provide complex carbs to fuel your day.

This burrito makes for a satisfying, balanced breakfast that can be enjoyed on the go. Pair it with a side of fresh fruit or a small serving of plain Greek yogurt for an even more well•rounded meal.

74. Low•Carb Muffins with Blueberries

Ingredient:

• 1 1/4 cups almond flour
• 1/4 cup coconut flour
• 1 tsp baking powder
• 1/4 tsp salt
• 3 large eggs
• 1/4 cup unsweetened almond milk
• 2 tbsp granulated erythritol or monk fruit sweetener
• 1 tsp vanilla extract
• 3/4 cup fresh or frozen blueberries

Instructions:

1. Preheat oven to 350°F. Grease a 12•cup muffin tin or line with paper liners.

2. In a medium bowl, whisk together the almond flour, coconut flour, baking powder, and salt.

3. In a separate bowl, beat the eggs. Then stir in the almond milk, erythritol/monk fruit, and vanilla.

4. Pour the wet ingredients into the dry ingredients and mix just until combined. Fold in the blueberries.

5. Scoop the batter evenly into the prepared muffin cups, filling them about 3/4 full.

6. Bake for 18•22 minutes, until a toothpick inserted in the center comes out clean.

7. Allow the muffins to cool in the pan for 5 minutes before transferring to a wire rack.

These low•carb blueberry muffins are a great diabetic•friendly baked good. The combination of almond flour and coconut flour keeps the carb count low, while the blueberries add natural sweetness and antioxidants.

The erythritol or monk fruit sweetener provides a touch of sweetness without spiking blood sugar. These muffins are moist, flavorful, and satisfying.

Enjoy these muffins as a snack or light breakfast. They pair well with a cup of unsweetened tea or coffee. This recipe makes a dozen muffins, so you can have them on hand throughout the week.

75. Green Smoothie with Spinach and Avocado

Ingredient:

- 1 cup unsweetened almond milk
- 1 cup packed fresh spinach leaves
- 1/2 avocado, pitted and peeled
- 1/2 cup frozen blueberries
- 1 tbsp ground flaxseed
- 1 tsp honey (optional)
- 1/2 tsp vanilla extract
- 1/4 tsp ground cinnamon

Instructions:

1. Add all the ingredients to a high·powered blender. Blend on high speed until completely smooth and creamy.

2. Pour the green smoothie into a glass and enjoy immediately.

Nutritional Info (per serving):
- Calories: 220
- Total Carbs: 16g
- Fiber: 8g
- Net Carbs: 8g
- Protein: 5g
- Fat: 15g

This green smoothie is an excellent choice for diabetics over 50 for several reasons:

- Spinach is packed with vitamins, minerals, and antioxidants, but very low in carbs.
- Avocado provides healthy monounsaturated fats to help slow the absorption of carbs.
- Blueberries are a low·glycemic fruit that adds natural sweetness and fiber.
- Flaxseed and cinnamon may help improve insulin sensitivity.
- The unsweetened almond milk and optional honey keep the carb count in check.

The combination of nutrient·dense greens, healthy fats, fiber, and a touch of natural sweetness makes this a very diabetes·friendly smoothie. It's a great way to pack in a serving of vegetables and fruit.

Enjoy this green smoothie as a nutritious breakfast or snack. It's a simple, delicious way to support overall health and blood sugar management for diabetics over 50.

76. Egg Muffins with Veggies and Turkey Sausage

Ingredient:

• 8 large eggs
• 1/2 cup unsweetened almond milk
• 1/4 tsp salt
• 1/4 tsp black pepper
• 1 cup diced bell peppers
• 1/2 cup diced onions
• 1/2 cup diced mushrooms
• 1/2 cup diced turkey sausage (or cooked turkey bacon)
• 2 tbsp shredded cheddar cheese (optional)

Instructions:

1. Preheat oven to 350°F. Grease a 12•cup muffin tin.

2. In a large bowl, whisk together the eggs, almond milk, salt, and pepper.

3. Stir in the diced bell peppers, onions, mushrooms, and turkey sausage until well combined.

4. Divide the egg mixture evenly among the prepared muffin cups, filling each about 3/4 full.

5. If using, sprinkle the shredded cheddar cheese on top of the egg muffins.

6. Bake for 20•25 minutes, until the eggs are set and the tops are lightly golden.

7. Allow the egg muffins to cool in the pan for 5 minutes before removing.

These egg muffins are an excellent diabetic•friendly breakfast or snack option. The combination of protein•rich eggs, fiber•filled vegetables, and lean turkey sausage helps keep blood sugar levels stable.

The almond milk and optional cheese add creaminess without significantly increasing the carb content. You can customize the veggie mix to your preferences.

These portable egg muffins are easy to make ahead and reheat throughout the week. Pair them with a side of fresh fruit or a small serving of Greek yogurt for a complete, diabetes•friendly meal.

77. Steel•Cut Oats with Almond Butter and Banana

Ingredient:

- 1/2 cup steel•cut oats
- 1 1/2 cups unsweetened almond milk
- 1 tbsp almond butter
- 1/2 medium banana, sliced
- 1 tsp ground cinnamon
- 1 tbsp chopped walnuts (optional)

Instructions:

1. In a small saucepan, bring the almond milk to a boil over medium•high heat.

2. Stir in the steel•cut oats and reduce heat to low. Simmer for 15•20 minutes, stirring occasionally, until the oats are tender and creamy.

3. Remove the oatmeal from heat and stir in the almond butter until well combined.

4. Transfer the oatmeal to a bowl and top with the sliced banana, cinnamon, and chopped walnuts (if using).

Nutritional Info (per serving):
- Calories: 320
- Total Carbs: 37g
- Fiber: 7g
- Net Carbs: 30g
- Protein: 10g
- Fat: 15g

This steel•cut oats breakfast is an excellent choice for diabetics over 50 for several reasons:

- Steel•cut oats are a high•fiber, low•glycemic complex carb that helps stabilize blood sugar.
- Almond butter provides healthy fats and protein to slow carb absorption.
- Banana adds natural sweetness and fiber.
- Cinnamon may help improve insulin sensitivity.
- Walnuts offer additional healthy fats and fiber.

The combination of complex carbs, fiber, protein, and healthy fats makes this a very diabetes•friendly meal. It will provide sustained energy and help keep blood sugar levels stable.

78. Cinnamon and Vanilla Protein Pancakes

Ingredient:

• 1/2 cup oat flour
• 1/4 cup unflavored whey protein powder
• 1 tsp baking powder
• 1/2 tsp ground cinnamon
• 1/4 tsp salt
• 1 large egg
• 1/2 cup unsweetened almond milk
• 1 tsp vanilla extract
• 1 tbsp granulated erythritol or monk fruit sweetener (optional)

Instructions:

1. In a medium bowl, whisk together the oat flour, protein powder, baking powder, cinnamon and salt.

2. In a separate bowl, beat the egg. Then stir in the almond milk and vanilla extract (and erythritol/monk fruit if using).

3. Pour the wet ingredients into the dry ingredients and stir just until combined (do not overmix).

4. Heat a non•stick skillet or griddle over medium heat. Lightly grease the surface.

5. Scoop the batter by 1/4 cup portions onto the hot surface. Cook for 2•3 minutes per side, until golden brown.

6. Serve the protein pancakes warm, with your desired toppings like berries, nuts, or a drizzle of sugar•free syrup.

Nutritional Info (per 3 pancakes):
• Calories: 190
• Total Carbs: 16g
• Fiber: 3g
• Net Carbs: 13g
• Protein: 18g
• Fat: 6g

These protein•packed pancakes are a great diabetic•friendly breakfast option. The oat flour, protein powder, and cinnamon help slow the absorption of carbs to prevent blood sugar spikes. The vanilla and optional sweetener add flavor without much added sugar.

79. Apple Cinnamon Quinoa Breakfast Bowl

Ingredient:

- 1/2 cup cooked quinoa
- 1/2 cup unsweetened almond milk
- 1/2 medium apple, diced
- 1 tbsp chopped walnuts
- 1 tsp ground cinnamon
- 1 tsp honey (optional)

Instructions:

1. In a small bowl, combine the cooked quinoa and almond milk. Microwave for 1•2 minutes until warm.

2. Stir in the diced apple, walnuts, and cinnamon until well mixed.

3. If desired, drizzle the quinoa bowl with a small amount of honey for added sweetness. Serve the apple cinnamon quinoa breakfast bowl warm.

Nutritional Info (per serving):
- Calories: 220
- Total Carbs: 30g
- Fiber: 5g
- Net Carbs: 25g
- Protein: 6g
- Fat: 9g

This apple cinnamon quinoa breakfast bowl is an excellent diabetic•friendly option for those over 50. Here's why it's a great choice:

- Quinoa is a high•fiber, high•protein whole grain that helps stabilize blood sugar.
- Apples provide natural sweetness and fiber to slow carb absorption.
- Walnuts add healthy fats and crunch.
- Cinnamon may help improve insulin sensitivity.
- The optional honey provides just a touch of sweetness without spiking blood sugar.

The combination of complex carbs, fiber, protein, and healthy fats makes this a very satisfying and diabetes•friendly breakfast. It will provide sustained energy and help keep blood sugar levels stable.

This quinoa bowl can be easily customized to your taste preferences. Try adding other diced fruit, nuts, or a sprinkle of unsweetened coconut. Enjoy it as a warm, comforting start to your day.

80. Chickpea Flour Omelette with Veggies

Ingredient:

• 1/2 cup chickpea (garbanzo bean) flour
• 2 large eggs, beaten
• 1/4 cup unsweetened almond milk
• 1/4 tsp baking powder
• 1/4 tsp turmeric
• 1/4 tsp garlic powder
• 1/4 tsp salt
• 1/8 tsp black pepper
• 1 cup mixed chopped vegetables (such as spinach, bell peppers, onions, mushrooms)
• 1 tbsp olive oil

Instructions:

1. In a medium bowl, whisk together the chickpea flour, eggs, almond milk, baking powder, turmeric, garlic powder, salt, and pepper until smooth.

2. Fold the chopped vegetables into the batter.

3. Heat the olive oil in a non•stick skillet over medium heat.

4. Pour the batter into the skillet, spreading it out evenly. Cook for 2•3 minutes per side, until the omelette is set and lightly browned. Carefully slide the omelette onto a plate. Serve warm.

This chickpea flour omelette is a great diabetic•friendly breakfast or brunch option. Chickpea flour is high in protein and fiber, helping to slow the absorption of carbs. The addition of nutrient•dense vegetables makes it a well•rounded, satisfying meal.

The turmeric, garlic, and black pepper add flavor without any added sugars. You can customize the veggie fillings to your taste preferences.

Serve this omelette with a side of fresh fruit or a small green salad for a complete, diabetes•friendly meal. It's a tasty way to start your day with a balance of protein, fiber, and healthy fats.

81. Chickpea and Avocado Salad

Ingredient:

- 1 (15 oz) can chickpeas, rinsed and drained
- 1 ripe avocado, diced
- 1/4 cup diced red onion
- 2 tbsp chopped fresh cilantro
- 1 tbsp fresh lemon juice
- 1 tsp extra virgin olive oil
- 1/4 tsp ground cumin
- 1/4 tsp salt
- 1/8 tsp black pepper

Instructions:

1. In a medium bowl, gently toss together the chickpeas, diced avocado, red onion, and cilantro.

2. In a small bowl, whisk together the lemon juice, olive oil, cumin, salt, and pepper.

3. Pour the dressing over the chickpea•avocado mixture and toss to coat evenly.

4. Serve the chickpea and avocado salad chilled or at room temperature.

This chickpea and avocado salad is an excellent diabetic•friendly option for a few reasons:

- Chickpeas are a high•fiber, high•protein legume that helps stabilize blood sugar.
- Avocado provides healthy monounsaturated fats to slow carb absorption.
- The simple lemon•olive oil dressing adds flavor without added sugars.
- Onion and cilantro provide antioxidants and additional flavor.

The combination of plant•based protein, fiber, and healthy fats makes this salad very satisfying and blood sugar•friendly. It can be enjoyed as a light main dish or side salad.

This salad is also very versatile • you can customize it by adding other diced veggies, herbs, or a sprinkle of feta or Parmesan cheese. Serve it on a bed of greens or with whole grain crackers for a complete, diabetic•friendly meal.

82. Chicken Salad Lettuce Wraps

Ingredient:

• 2 cups cooked, shredded chicken breast
• 1/4 cup plain Greek yogurt
• 1 tbsp Dijon mustard
• 1 tbsp lemon juice
• 1/4 cup diced celery
• 2 tbsp diced red onion
• 1 tbsp chopped fresh parsley
• 1/4 tsp salt
• 1/8 tsp black pepper
• 8•10 large lettuce leaves (such as romaine or butter lettuce)

Instructions:

1. In a medium bowl, mix together the shredded chicken, Greek yogurt, Dijon mustard, lemon juice, celery, red onion, parsley, salt, and pepper until well combined.

2. Spoon the chicken salad mixture evenly into the lettuce leaves, creating lettuce wraps.

3. Serve the chicken salad lettuce wraps immediately.

These chicken salad lettuce wraps are an excellent diabetic•friendly option for a few reasons:

• Chicken is a lean protein that won't spike blood sugar.

• Greek yogurt provides protein and creaminess without added sugars.

• The vegetables add fiber, vitamins, and minerals.

• Lettuce leaves are low in carbs and calories, making them a great alternative to bread or tortillas.

The combination of protein, fiber, and healthy fats in this recipe helps keep blood sugar levels stable. It's a satisfying and nutritious meal or snack.

You can customize the chicken salad by adding other diced veggies, herbs, or a sprinkle of nuts or seeds. Serve the lettuce wraps with a side salad or some sliced cucumber for an even more well•rounded diabetic•friendly meal.

83. Egg Salad with Greek Yogurt

Ingredient:

- 6 hard•boiled eggs, peeled and chopped
- 1/2 cup plain, unsweetened Greek yogurt
- 1 tbsp Dijon mustard
- 1 tbsp chopped fresh dill (or 1 tsp dried dill)
- 2 tsp lemon juice
- 1/4 tsp salt
- 1/8 tsp black pepper

Instructions:

1. In a medium bowl, combine the chopped hard•boiled eggs, Greek yogurt, Dijon mustard, dill, lemon juice, salt, and pepper. Stir until well mixed.

2. Taste and adjust seasonings as needed. Serve the egg salad on a bed of lettuce, on whole grain crackers, or stuffed into celery sticks.

Nutritional Info (per 1/4 cup serving):
- Calories: 80
- Total Carbs: 2g
- Fiber: 0g
- Net Carbs: 2g
- Protein: 8g
- Fat: 5g

This egg salad made with Greek yogurt is an excellent diabetic•friendly option for a few reasons:

- Eggs are a high•quality, protein•rich food that won't spike blood sugar.
- Greek yogurt provides creaminess and additional protein without added sugars.
- The Dijon mustard, dill, and lemon juice add flavor without needing to use high•carb ingredients like mayonnaise.

The combination of protein, healthy fats, and minimal carbs makes this egg salad very diabetes•friendly. It's a satisfying and nutritious option for a snack or light meal.

You can enjoy the egg salad on its own, on top of greens, or with low•carb crackers or veggie sticks. It's a versatile dish that can be customized to your taste preferences.

This recipe is a great way for diabetics to get the benefits of eggs in a tasty, blood sugar•friendly preparation.

84. Quinoa and Black Bean Stuffed Peppers

Ingredient:

• 4 medium bell peppers, halved lengthwise and seeds removed
• 1 cup cooked quinoa
• 1 (15 oz) can black beans, rinsed and drained
• 1/2 cup diced tomatoes
• 1/4 cup diced onion
• 2 cloves garlic, minced
• 1 tsp ground cumin
• 1/2 tsp chili powder
• 1/4 tsp salt
• 1/4 tsp black pepper
• 1/2 cup shredded low•fat cheddar or Monterey Jack cheese

Instructions:

1. Preheat oven to 375°F. Arrange the bell pepper halves in a baking dish.

2. In a medium bowl, combine the cooked quinoa, black beans, diced tomatoes, onion, garlic, cumin, chili powder, salt, and pepper. Stir to mix well.

3. Spoon the quinoa•black bean mixture evenly into the bell pepper halves.

4. Top each stuffed pepper with a sprinkle of shredded cheese.

5. Bake for 25•30 minutes, until the peppers are tender and the filling is hot.

6. Serve the stuffed peppers warm.

These quinoa and black bean stuffed peppers are an excellent diabetic•friendly meal. The combination of high•fiber quinoa, protein•rich black beans, and nutrient•dense bell peppers makes for a balanced, low•carb dish.

The spices add flavor without added sugars. The cheese topping provides a creamy, satisfying element. This recipe is easy to prepare and can be enjoyed as a main dish or side.

Stuffed peppers are a great way for diabetics to enjoy a hearty, diabetes•friendly meal. Pair it with a fresh salad for a complete, well•rounded dinner.

85. Grilled Vegetable and Hummus Wrap

Ingredient:

- 1 zucchini, sliced lengthwise into 1/4•inch thick strips
- 1 red bell pepper, sliced into strips
- 1 yellow squash, sliced lengthwise into 1/4•inch thick strips
- 1 eggplant, sliced lengthwise into 1/4•inch thick strips
- 2 tbsp olive oil
- Salt and pepper to taste
- 4 whole wheat tortillas or wraps
- 1 cup hummus
- 1 cup baby spinach or arugula

Instructions:

1. Preheat grill or grill pan to medium•high heat.

2. Toss the sliced zucchini, bell pepper, yellow squash, and eggplant with the olive oil. Season with salt and pepper.

3. Grill the vegetables for 2•3 minutes per side, until tender and charred in spots. Remove from grill and let cool slightly.

4. Spread about 1/4 cup of hummus onto each tortilla or wrap, leaving a 1•inch border.

5. Arrange the grilled vegetables in a line down the center of each wrap. Top with a handful of baby spinach or arugula.

6. Fold the bottom of the wrap up over the filling, then fold in the sides and continue rolling up tightly.

7. Slice the wraps in half diagonally and serve.

These grilled vegetable and hummus wraps make a delicious, nutritious, and portable lunch or snack. The combination of the flavorful grilled veggies, creamy hummus, and fresh greens is so satisfying. Enjoy!

86. Zoodle Salad with Pesto and Cherry Tomatoes

Ingredient:

• 3 medium zucchinis, spiralized into zoodles
• 1 cup cherry tomatoes, halved
• 1/2 cup basil pesto (store•bought or homemade)
• 2 tbsp toasted pine nuts
• 2 tbsp grated Parmesan cheese
• Salt and pepper to taste

Instructions:

1. In a large bowl, combine the spiralized zucchini noodles and halved cherry tomatoes.

2. Add the basil pesto and toss gently to coat the zoodles evenly.

3. Sprinkle the toasted pine nuts and grated Parmesan cheese over the top.

4. Season with salt and pepper to taste.

5. Serve immediately or refrigerate until ready to serve.

This zoodle salad is a fresh, flavorful, and low•carb option. The zucchini noodles provide a pasta•like texture, while the pesto, tomatoes, pine nuts, and Parmesan add tons of flavor.

It's a great option for a light lunch or side dish. The pesto and vegetables provide fiber, vitamins, and antioxidants, making it a nutritious choice.

You can use store•bought pesto or make your own homemade version. Adjust the amount of pesto to your taste preference. Enjoy this delicious and healthy zoodle salad!

87. Chicken and Kale Salad with Balsamic Dressing

Ingredient:

- 4 cups chopped kale
- 1 cup cooked, shredded chicken breast
- 1/2 cup cherry tomatoes, halved
- 1/4 cup sliced cucumber
- 2 tbsp crumbled feta cheese
- 2 tbsp toasted slivered almonds

Balsamic Dressing:

- 2 tbsp balsamic vinegar
- 1 tbsp olive oil
- 1 tsp Dijon mustard
- 1 tsp honey
- 1 garlic clove, minced
- Salt and pepper to taste

Instructions:

1. In a large salad bowl, combine the chopped kale, shredded chicken, cherry tomatoes, cucumber, feta cheese, and toasted almonds.

2. In a small bowl, whisk together the balsamic vinegar, olive oil, Dijon mustard, honey, and minced garlic. Season with salt and pepper.

3. Drizzle the balsamic dressing over the salad and toss gently to coat.

4. Serve immediately.

This salad is packed with nutrient•dense kale, lean protein from the chicken, and healthy fats from the olive oil and almonds. The balsamic dressing provides a flavorful, low•sugar way to dress the salad.

The portion sizes and ingredients make this a great option for a diabetic•friendly meal after 50. The fiber, protein, and healthy fats will help keep blood sugar levels stable.

88. Greek Salad with Feta and Olives

Ingredient:

• 5 cups chopped romaine lettuce
• 1 cup diced cucumber
• 1/2 cup halved cherry tomatoes
• 1/4 cup crumbled feta cheese
• 1/4 cup pitted kalamata olives, halved
• 2 tbsp red onion, thinly sliced
• 2 tbsp olive oil
• 1 tbsp red wine vinegar
• 1 tsp dried oregano
• 1/4 tsp salt
• 1/8 tsp black pepper

Instructions:

1. In a large salad bowl, combine the chopped romaine, cucumber, cherry tomatoes, feta, olives, and red onion.

2. In a small bowl, whisk together the olive oil, red wine vinegar, oregano, salt, and pepper to make the dressing.

3. Drizzle the dressing over the salad and toss gently to coat.

This Greek salad is an excellent choice for diabetics over 50 for several reasons:

• Romaine lettuce and other vegetables provide fiber, vitamins, and minerals without many carbs.
• Feta cheese is a source of protein and healthy fats.
• Olives add more healthy fats and antioxidants.
• The olive oil and vinegar dressing is low in carbs and high in anti•inflammatory compounds.

The combination of nutrient•dense veggies, protein, and healthy fats helps keep blood sugar levels stable. This salad is very satisfying and can be enjoyed as a main dish or side.

You can customize the salad by adding grilled chicken or chickpeas for extra protein. Pair it with a small portion of whole grain crackers or a slice of sourdough bread for a more complete meal.

This Greek salad is a refreshing, diabetes•friendly option that's perfect for those over 50.

89. Soba Noodle Salad with Edamame and Carrots

Ingredient:

- 8 oz soba noodles
- 1 cup shelled edamame
- 2 carrots, julienned or grated
- 3 green onions, sliced
- 1/4 cup rice vinegar
- 2 tbsp soy sauce
- 1 tbsp sesame oil
- 1 tsp honey
- 1 tsp grated ginger
- 1 tsp sesame seeds
- Salt and pepper to taste

Instructions:

1. Cook the soba noodles according to package instructions. Drain and rinse under cold water.

2. In a large bowl, combine the cooked soba noodles, edamame, carrots, and green onions.

3. In a small bowl, whisk together the rice vinegar, soy sauce, sesame oil, honey, and grated ginger.

4. Pour the dressing over the noodle salad and toss to coat evenly.

5. Sprinkle the sesame seeds over the top and season with salt and pepper to taste.

6. Refrigerate for at least 30 minutes to allow the flavors to meld. Serve chilled or at room temperature.

Enjoy this refreshing and flavorful soba noodle salad! The combination of the nutty soba noodles, crunchy vegetables, and tangy•sweet dressing makes for a delicious and healthy meal.

9O. Tuna and White Bean Salad

Ingredient:

• 1 (15 oz) can white beans, drained and rinsed
• 1 (5 oz) can tuna, drained
• 1/2 cup diced celery
• 1/4 cup diced red onion
• 2 tbsp chopped fresh parsley
• 2 tbsp lemon juice
• 1 tbsp olive oil
• 1 tsp Dijon mustard
• Salt and pepper to taste

Instructions:

1. In a medium bowl, gently combine the drained and rinsed white beans, drained tuna, diced celery, diced red onion, and chopped parsley.

2. In a small bowl, whisk together the lemon juice, olive oil, and Dijon mustard. Season with salt and pepper.

3. Pour the dressing over the tuna and bean mixture and toss gently to coat.

4. Refrigerate the salad for at least 30 minutes to allow the flavors to meld.

5. Serve chilled or at room temperature. Can be served on a bed of greens, with whole grain crackers, or on its own.

This tuna and white bean salad is a simple, protein•packed dish that makes a great lunch or light dinner. The combination of tuna, white beans, vegetables, and a tangy dressing creates a satisfying and nutritious meal.

The white beans provide fiber and complex carbs, while the tuna adds lean protein. This salad is also low in calories and fat, making it a great option for a healthy diet.

Adjust the amounts of ingredients to your taste preferences. Enjoy this easy and flavorful tuna and white bean salad!

91. Chicken and Cauliflower Rice Pilaf

Ingredient:

• 1 lb boneless, skinless chicken breasts, cubed
• 1 tbsp olive oil
• 1 cup diced onion
• 2 cloves garlic, minced
• 1 cup riced cauliflower
• 1/2 cup diced bell pepper
• 1/4 cup sliced green onions
• 2 tbsp chopped fresh parsley
• 1 tsp ground cumin
• 1/4 tsp salt
• 1/8 tsp black pepper

Instructions:

1. In a large skillet, heat the olive oil over medium•high heat. Add the cubed chicken and cook for 5•7 minutes, until no longer pink. Remove the chicken from the skillet and set aside.

2. In the same skillet, sauté the diced onion for 3•4 minutes until translucent. Add the minced garlic and cook for 1 minute more.

3. Stir in the riced cauliflower, diced bell pepper, sliced green onions, parsley, cumin, salt, and pepper. Cook for 5•7 minutes, until the cauliflower is tender.

4. Return the cooked chicken to the skillet and toss everything together until well combined and heated through. Serve the chicken and cauliflower rice pilaf warm.

This chicken and cauliflower rice pilaf is an excellent diabetic•friendly dish for several reasons:

• Cauliflower rice is a low•carb, high•fiber alternative to traditional rice.
• Chicken is a lean protein that won't spike blood sugar levels.
• The vegetables provide fiber, vitamins, and antioxidants.
• The simple seasoning of cumin, salt, and pepper adds flavor without added sugars.

The combination of protein, fiber, and minimal carbs helps keep blood sugar stable. This makes it a great option for diabetics.

You can customize the dish by adding other diced vegetables, fresh herbs, or a sprinkle of nuts or seeds. Serve it as a main course or alongside a fresh salad for a complete, diabetes•friendly meal.

92. Seared Scallops with Asparagus and Lemon Butter

Ingredient:

- 1 lb sea scallops, patted dry
- 1 tbsp olive oil
- 1 lb asparagus, trimmed and cut into 1•inch pieces
- 2 tbsp unsalted butter
- 2 tbsp freshly squeezed lemon juice
- 1 tsp grated lemon zest
- 2 tbsp chopped fresh parsley
- Salt and pepper to taste

Instructions:

1. Season the scallops with salt and pepper.

2. Heat the olive oil in a large skillet over medium•high heat. When the oil is hot, add the scallops in a single layer and sear for 2•3 minutes per side, until golden brown. Transfer the seared scallops to a plate.

3. In the same skillet, add the asparagus pieces and a splash of water. Cover and cook for 3•5 minutes, until the asparagus is tender•crisp.

4. Reduce the heat to low and add the butter, lemon juice, and lemon zest to the skillet. Stir until the butter is melted and the sauce is combined.

5. Return the seared scallops to the skillet and gently toss to coat with the lemon butter sauce.

6. Sprinkle the chopped parsley over the top.

7. Serve the seared scallops and asparagus immediately, spooning any extra lemon butter sauce over the top.

This dish features tender, seared scallops paired with crisp•tender asparagus in a bright, lemony butter sauce. It's a simple yet elegant meal that's perfect for a special occasion or weeknight dinner.

The combination of the sweet scallops, fresh asparagus, and tangy lemon butter creates a delicious and well•balanced flavor profile. Enjoy this healthy and flavorful seafood dish!

93. Turkey and Spinach Stuffed Peppers

Ingredient:

- 4 bell peppers, halved lengthwise and seeds removed
- 1 lb ground turkey
- 1 cup cooked brown rice
- 2 cups baby spinach, chopped
- 1/2 cup diced onion
- 2 garlic cloves, minced
- 1 tsp dried oregano
- 1/2 tsp dried basil
- 1/4 tsp red pepper flakes (optional)
- 1 cup shredded mozzarella cheese
- Salt and pepper to taste

Instructions:

1. Preheat oven to 375°F.

2. In a large skillet, cook the ground turkey over medium heat until browned and cooked through, 5•7 minutes. Drain any excess fat.

3. Add the onion and garlic to the skillet and cook for 2•3 minutes until softened.

4. Stir in the cooked brown rice, chopped spinach, oregano, basil, and red pepper flakes (if using). Season with salt and pepper.

5. Arrange the bell pepper halves in a baking dish. Stuff each pepper half evenly with the turkey and spinach mixture.

6. Top the stuffed peppers with the shredded mozzarella cheese.

7. Bake for 20•25 minutes, until the peppers are tender and the cheese is melted and bubbly.

8. Serve the stuffed peppers hot.

These turkey and spinach stuffed peppers are a healthy and delicious meal. The lean ground turkey, nutrient•rich spinach, and whole grain brown rice make it a balanced and satisfying dish. The melted cheese on top adds a nice creamy element. Enjoy!

94. Beef and Vegetable Kabobs

Ingredient:

• 1 lb beef sirloin or tenderloin, cut into 1•inch cubes
• 1 red bell pepper, cut into 1•inch pieces
• 1 yellow bell pepper, cut into 1•inch pieces
• 1 zucchini, cut into 1•inch slices
• 1 red onion, cut into 1•inch pieces
• 8 oz mushrooms, halved
• 2 tbsp olive oil
• 2 tbsp balsamic vinegar
• 1 tsp dried oregano
• 1 tsp garlic powder
• Salt and pepper to taste

Instructions:

1. In a large bowl, combine the beef cubes, bell pepper pieces, zucchini slices, onion pieces, and mushrooms.

2. In a small bowl, whisk together the olive oil, balsamic vinegar, oregano, garlic powder, salt, and pepper.

3. Pour the marinade over the beef and vegetables and toss to coat everything evenly. Cover and refrigerate for at least 30 minutes, up to 2 hours.

4. Preheat grill or grill pan to medium•high heat.

5. Thread the marinated beef and vegetables onto skewers, alternating the ingredients.

6. Grill the kabobs for 10•12 minutes, turning occasionally, until the beef is cooked through and the vegetables are tender.

7. Serve the beef and vegetable kabobs immediately, with any remaining marinade drizzled over the top.

Enjoy your delicious and healthy grilled kabobs!

95. Spaghetti Squash Primavera

Ingredient:

- 1 medium spaghetti squash, halved and seeded
- 1 tbsp olive oil
- 1 cup diced zucchini
- 1 cup diced bell peppers
- 1/2 cup diced onion
- 2 cloves garlic, minced
- 1 cup cherry tomatoes, halved
- 1/4 cup grated Parmesan cheese
- 2 tbsp chopped fresh basil
- 1 tbsp lemon juice
- 1/4 tsp salt
- 1/8 tsp black pepper

Instructions:

1. Preheat oven to 400°F. Place the spaghetti squash halves cut•side down on a baking sheet. Roast for 30•40 minutes, until tender when pierced with a fork.

2. In a large skillet, heat the olive oil over medium heat. Add the zucchini, bell peppers, onion, and garlic. Sauté for 5•7 minutes, until the vegetables are tender.

3. Use a fork to scrape the spaghetti squash flesh into strands, creating "noodles". Add the spaghetti squash noodles to the skillet with the sautéed vegetables.

4. Stir in the cherry tomatoes, Parmesan cheese, basil, lemon juice, salt, and pepper. Toss everything together until well combined. Serve the spaghetti squash primavera warm.

This spaghetti squash primavera is an excellent diabetic•friendly dish for a few reasons:

- Spaghetti squash is a low•carb, high•fiber vegetable that makes a great pasta alternative.
- The colorful mix of vegetables provides fiber, vitamins, and antioxidants.
- Parmesan cheese adds protein and healthy fats without much carbohydrate.
- Lemon juice and fresh basil provide flavor without added sugars.

The combination of fiber, protein, and healthy fats helps slow the absorption of carbs, keeping blood sugar levels stable. This makes it a great option for diabetics over 50. Serve this spaghetti squash primavera as a main dish or side. It pairs well with grilled chicken or shrimp for a complete, diabetes•friendly meal.

96. Chicken and Vegetable Kebabs

Ingredient:

• 1 lb boneless, skinless chicken breasts, cut into 1•inch cubes
• 1 red bell pepper, cut into 1•inch pieces
• 1 yellow bell pepper, cut into 1•inch pieces
• 1 zucchini, cut into 1•inch slices
• 1 red onion, cut into 1•inch pieces
• 8 oz mushrooms, halved
• 2 tbsp olive oil
• 2 tbsp balsamic vinegar
• 1 tsp dried oregano
• 1 tsp garlic powder
• 1/4 tsp salt
• 1/4 tsp black pepper

Instructions:

1. In a large bowl, combine the chicken cubes, bell pepper pieces, zucchini slices, onion pieces, and mushrooms.

2. In a small bowl, whisk together the olive oil, balsamic vinegar, oregano, garlic powder, salt, and pepper.

3. Pour the marinade over the chicken and vegetables and toss to coat everything evenly. Cover and refrigerate for at least 30 minutes, up to 2 hours.

4. Preheat grill or grill pan to medium•high heat.

5. Thread the marinated chicken and vegetables onto skewers, alternating the ingredients.

6. Grill the kebabs for 12•15 minutes, turning occasionally, until the chicken is cooked through and the vegetables are tender.

7. Serve the chicken and vegetable kebabs immediately.

This recipe is diabetic•friendly, as it is low in carbs and provides a balance of lean protein, vegetables, and healthy fats. The marinade adds flavor without adding too many additional calories or carbs. Enjoy this delicious and nutritious grilled kebab dish!

97. Vegetable and Chickpea Curry

Ingredient:

- 1 tbsp olive oil
- 1 onion, diced
- 3 cloves garlic, minced
- 1 tbsp grated fresh ginger
- 2 tsp curry powder
- 1 tsp ground cumin
- 1/2 tsp ground coriander
- 1/4 tsp cayenne pepper (or to taste)
- 1 cup diced tomatoes (fresh or canned, no•salt•added)
- 1 cup low•sodium vegetable broth
- 1 (15 oz) can chickpeas, rinsed and drained
- 1 medium cauliflower, cut into florets
- 1 medium zucchini, diced
- 1 cup frozen peas
- 1/4 cup chopped fresh cilantro
- Salt and black pepper to taste

Instructions:

1. In a large skillet or Dutch oven, heat the olive oil over medium heat. Add the onion and sauté for 3•4 minutes, until translucent.

2. Add the garlic and ginger and sauté for 1 minute, until fragrant.

3. Stir in the curry powder, cumin, coriander, and cayenne. Cook for 1 minute to toast the spices.

4. Add the diced tomatoes, vegetable broth, chickpeas, cauliflower, zucchini, and frozen peas. Bring the mixture to a simmer.

5. Reduce the heat to low, cover, and let the curry simmer for 15•20 minutes, or until the vegetables are tender.

6. Remove from heat and stir in the chopped cilantro. Season with salt and black pepper to taste.

This Vegetable and Chickpea Curry is a delicious and diabetic•friendly dish. The combination of vegetables, chickpeas, and aromatic spices provides a flavorful and nutrient•dense meal. The high fiber content from the chickpeas and vegetables helps to regulate blood sugar levels.

98. Baked Chicken Parmesan with Zoodles

Ingredient:

• 4 boneless, skinless chicken breasts
• 1/2 cup whole wheat breadcrumbs
• 1/4 cup grated Parmesan cheese
• 1 tsp dried oregano
• 1/2 tsp garlic powder
• 1/4 tsp salt
• 1/4 tsp black pepper
• 1 cup marinara sauce (no•sugar•added)
• 1/2 cup shredded part•skim mozzarella cheese
• 3 medium zucchinis, spiralized into "zoodles"
• 2 tbsp olive oil

Instructions:

1. Preheat your oven to 400°F (200°C). Lightly grease a baking sheet or use a nonstick baking mat.

2. In a shallow bowl, combine the breadcrumbs, Parmesan cheese, oregano, garlic powder, salt, and pepper.

3. Dip the chicken breasts in the breadcrumb mixture, pressing gently to help the coating adhere.

4. Place the breaded chicken on the prepared baking sheet. Bake for 20•25 minutes, or until the chicken is cooked through and the breading is golden brown.

5. Remove the chicken from the oven and top each piece with 1/4 cup of marinara sauce and 2 tablespoons of mozzarella cheese.

6. Return the chicken to the oven and bake for an additional 5•7 minutes, or until the cheese is melted and bubbly.

7. While the chicken is baking, heat the olive oil in a large skillet over medium heat. Add the spiralized zucchini "zoodles" and sauté for 3•5 minutes, or until they are tender but still have a slight crunch. Serve the baked chicken parmesan on top of the sautéed zoodles.

This Baked Chicken Parmesan with Zoodles is a diabetic•friendly dish that is low in carbs and high in protein and fiber. The zucchini noodles provide a healthy, low•carb alternative to traditional pasta, while the baked chicken parmesan adds a satisfying and flavorful protein source.

99. Garlic Shrimp and Broccoli Stir•Fry

Ingredient:

- 1 lb peeled and deveined shrimp
- 2 tbsp low•sodium soy sauce
- 1 tbsp rice vinegar
- 1 tsp sesame oil
- 2 tsp cornstarch
- 2 tbsp olive oil
- 4 cloves garlic, minced
- 1 lb broccoli florets
- 1/2 cup low•sodium chicken or vegetable broth
- 1 tsp grated fresh ginger
- 1/4 tsp red pepper flakes (optional)
- Salt and black pepper to taste

Instructions:

1. In a medium bowl, combine the shrimp, soy sauce, rice vinegar, sesame oil, and cornstarch. Toss to coat the shrimp and set aside.

2. Heat the olive oil in a large skillet or wok over medium•high heat. Add the minced garlic and sauté for 1 minute, until fragrant.

3. Add the broccoli florets to the skillet and stir•fry for 2•3 minutes, until the broccoli starts to soften.

4. Add the marinated shrimp and the broth to the skillet. Bring the mixture to a simmer and cook for 3•5 minutes, or until the shrimp are cooked through and the broccoli is tender•crisp.

5. Stir in the grated ginger and red pepper flakes (if using). Season with salt and black pepper to taste.

6. Serve the garlic shrimp and broccoli stir•fry immediately, over cauliflower rice or steamed quinoa, if desired.

This Garlic Shrimp and Broccoli Stir•Fry is a diabetic•friendly meal that is high in protein, low in carbs, and packed with fiber and nutrients. The shrimp provides a lean source of protein, while the broccoli adds essential vitamins, minerals, and antioxidants.

The stir•fry is quick and easy to prepare, making it a great option for a weeknight dinner. Serve it over a bed of cauliflower rice or steamed quinoa for a complete and satisfying diabetic•friendly meal.

100. Lamb and Vegetable Stew

Ingredient:

• 1 lb lean lamb, cut into 1•inch cubes
• 2 tbsp olive oil
• 1 onion, diced
• 3 cloves garlic, minced
• 2 carrots, peeled and sliced
• 2 celery stalks, sliced
• 1 cup diced tomatoes (fresh or canned, no•salt•added)
• 2 cups low•sodium beef or chicken broth
• 1 tsp dried thyme
• 1 tsp dried rosemary
• 1/2 tsp salt
• 1/4 tsp black pepper
• 1 cup cubed zucchini
• 1 cup green beans, trimmed and cut into 1•inch pieces

Instructions:

1. In a large pot or Dutch oven, heat the olive oil over medium•high heat. Add the lamb cubes and brown on all sides, about 5 minutes total. Remove the lamb from the pot and set aside.

2. Add the onion and garlic to the pot and sauté for 2•3 minutes, until fragrant and translucent.

3. Add the carrots, celery, tomatoes, broth, thyme, rosemary, salt, and pepper. Bring the mixture to a boil, then reduce the heat and let it simmer for 15 minutes.

4. Add the cooked lamb, zucchini, and green beans to the pot. Simmer for an additional 15•20 minutes, or until the vegetables are tender and the lamb is cooked through.

5. Taste and adjust seasoning as needed.

This lamb and vegetable stew is a diabetic•friendly meal that is high in protein, low in carbs, and packed with fiber and nutrients from the vegetables. The lean lamb provides a satisfying source of protein, while the vegetables add essential vitamins, minerals, and antioxidants.

Enjoy this comforting and healthy stew as a main dish or serve it with a side salad for a complete diabetic•friendly meal.

101. Yogurt with Flaxseeds and Berries

Ingredient:

- 1 cup plain Greek yogurt (full•fat or low•fat)
- 2 tbsp ground flaxseeds
- 1 cup mixed berries (such as blueberries, raspberries, and/or blackberries)
- 1 tsp honey (optional)

Instructions:

1. In a medium bowl, combine the plain Greek yogurt and ground flaxseeds. Stir until well mixed.

2. Top the yogurt mixture with the mixed berries.

3. If desired, drizzle the honey over the top of the berries.

Nutritional Information (per serving):
Calories: 180
Total Carbs: 16g
Fiber: 5g
Net Carbs: 11g
Protein: 15g
Fat: 7g

This Yogurt with Flaxseeds and Berries is a delicious and diabetic•friendly snack or breakfast option. The Greek yogurt provides a good source of protein, while the flaxseeds add fiber, healthy fats, and additional nutrients.

The mixed berries are a low•glycemic fruit that are high in antioxidants and fiber, helping to regulate blood sugar levels. The optional honey can add a touch of sweetness, but it can be omitted if you prefer a less sweet version.

This recipe is easy to prepare and can be enjoyed as a quick and nutritious snack or part of a balanced diabetic•friendly meal. The combination of protein, fiber, and healthy fats will help keep you feeling full and satisfied.

Enjoy this Yogurt with Flaxseeds and Berries as a delicious and diabetic•friendly treat!

102. Almond Flour Crackers with Cheese

Ingredient:

• 1 1/2 cups almond flour
• 1/4 cup grated Parmesan cheese
• 1/4 cup shredded cheddar cheese
• 1 tsp dried thyme
• 1/2 tsp garlic powder
• 1/4 tsp salt
• 2 tbsp unsalted butter, melted
• 1 tbsp water

Instructions:

1. Preheat your oven to 350°F (175°C). Line a baking sheet with parchment paper.

2. In a medium bowl, combine the almond flour, Parmesan cheese, cheddar cheese, thyme, garlic powder, and salt. Mix well.

3. Add the melted butter and water to the dry ingredients. Stir until a dough forms.

4. Roll the dough out between two sheets of parchment paper to about 1/8•inch thickness.

5. Use a sharp knife or cookie cutter to cut the dough into cracker shapes.

6. Carefully transfer the crackers to the prepared baking sheet, spacing them apart.

7. Bake for 12•15 minutes, or until the crackers are golden brown and crispy.

8. Remove the crackers from the oven and let them cool completely on the baking sheet before serving.

These Almond Flour Crackers with Cheese are a delicious and diabetic•friendly snack or appetizer. The almond flour provides a low•carb, high•fiber base, while the Parmesan and cheddar cheeses add flavor and a satisfying crunch.

These crackers are perfect for dipping in hummus, serving with a cheese plate, or enjoying on their own as a healthy snack. They are a great option for those following a diabetic diet after 50, as they are low in carbs and high in healthy fats and protein.

Enjoy these tasty and nutritious Almond Flour Crackers with Cheese as part of your diabetic•friendly diet.

1O3. Fresh Berries with Whipped Cream

Ingredient:

- 1 cup mixed fresh berries (such as strawberries, raspberries, blueberries)
- 1/2 cup heavy whipping cream
- 1 tbsp powdered erythritol or other low•calorie sweetener
- 1/2 tsp vanilla extract

Instructions:

1. In a medium bowl, combine the heavy whipping cream, powdered erythritol, and vanilla extract. Using a hand mixer or stand mixer, whip the cream until it forms soft peaks.

2. Gently fold the whipped cream into the fresh berries, being careful not to crush the berries.

3. Serve the fresh berries with whipped cream immediately, or chill in the refrigerator for up to 30 minutes before serving.

Nutritional Information (per serving):
Calories: 120
Total Carbs: 8g
Fiber: 3g
Net Carbs: 5g
Protein: 2g
Fat: 9g

This Fresh Berries with Whipped Cream is a delightful and diabetic•friendly dessert or snack. The combination of fresh, low•glycemic berries and lightly sweetened whipped cream provides a satisfying and nutrient•dense treat.

The heavy whipping cream is a good source of healthy fats, while the berries are high in fiber and antioxidants. The powdered erythritol, a low•calorie sweetener, helps to keep the carb and sugar content low, making this a suitable option for those following a diabetic diet after 50.

This dessert is easy to prepare and can be enjoyed as a light and refreshing treat. It's a great way to incorporate more fresh fruits into your diabetic•friendly diet.

Enjoy this Fresh Berries with Whipped Cream as a delicious and nutritious dessert or snack!

104. Sliced Bell Peppers with Salsa

Ingredient:

• 2 large bell peppers (any color), sliced into strips
• 1 cup fresh salsa (or low•sodium, low•sugar store•bought salsa)
• 2 tbsp crumbled feta cheese (optional)
• 1 tbsp chopped fresh cilantro (optional)

Instructions:

1. Wash the bell peppers and slice them into long, thin strips.

2. Arrange the bell pepper strips on a serving platter or plate.

3. Top the bell pepper strips with the fresh salsa, spreading it evenly over the peppers.

4. If desired, sprinkle the crumbled feta cheese and chopped fresh cilantro over the top.

Nutritional Information (per serving, without feta or cilantro):
Calories: 45
Total Carbs: 9g
Fiber: 3g
Net Carbs: 6g
Protein: 1g
Fat: 0g

This recipe is an excellent diabetic•friendly snack or appetizer. The bell peppers provide a crunchy, low•carb base, while the salsa adds flavor and a touch of natural sweetness without added sugars. The optional feta cheese and cilantro can provide additional flavor and nutrients.

This dish is high in fiber, low in calories and carbs, and rich in vitamins and antioxidants from the bell peppers and salsa. It's a great way to incorporate more vegetables into your diet while satisfying your taste buds.

Enjoy this refreshing and healthy Sliced Bell Peppers with Salsa as a snack or side dish for a diabetic•friendly meal.

105. Raw Veggies with Baba Ganoush

Ingredient:

Baba Ganoush:
- 1 medium eggplant
- 2 tbsp tahini
- 2 tbsp fresh lemon juice
- 2 cloves garlic, minced
- 1/4 tsp ground cumin
- 1/4 tsp salt
- 2 tbsp extra•virgin olive oil

Veggie Platter:
- 1 cup baby carrots
- 1 cup cucumber slices
- 1 cup cherry tomatoes
- 1 cup bell pepper strips (any color)
- 1 cup celery sticks

Instructions:

Baba Ganoush:

1. Preheat your oven to 400°F (200°C).

2. Pierce the eggplant several times with a fork. Roast the eggplant directly on the oven rack for 30•40 minutes, or until very soft.

3. Allow the eggplant to cool slightly, then cut it in half and scoop out the flesh into a food processor.

4. Add the tahini, lemon juice, garlic, cumin, and salt to the food processor. Blend until smooth.

5. Drizzle the olive oil over the baba ganoush and stir to combine.

Veggie Platter:

1. Arrange the raw vegetables (carrots, cucumber, tomatoes, bell pepper, and celery) on a serving platter.

2. Serve the baba ganoush alongside the raw veggies for dipping.

This Raw Veggies with Baba Ganoush is a delicious and diabetic•friendly snack or appetizer. The baba ganoush, a creamy eggplant•based dip, provides a flavorful and nutrient•dense option for dipping the fresh, crunchy vegetables.

The combination of the low•carb, high•fiber vegetables and the healthy fats from the tahini and olive oil in the baba ganoush makes this a great choice for a diabetic diet after 50. The fiber and nutrients from the vegetables can help regulate blood sugar levels and promote overall health.

106. Roasted Pumpkin Seeds with Sea Salt

Ingredient:
• 1 cup raw pumpkin seeds (also known as pepitas)
• 1 tsp olive oil
• 1/4 tsp sea salt

Instructions:
1. Preheat your oven to 325°F (165°C). Line a baking sheet with parchment paper.

2. In a small bowl, toss the raw pumpkin seeds with the olive oil until they are evenly coated.

3. Spread the pumpkin seeds in a single layer on the prepared baking sheet.

4. Sprinkle the sea salt evenly over the pumpkin seeds.

5. Roast the pumpkin seeds for 15•20 minutes, stirring halfway, until they are lightly golden and crispy.

6. Remove the roasted pumpkin seeds from the oven and let them cool completely before serving.

Nutritional Information (per serving, about 1/4 cup):
Calories: 90
Total Carbs: 3g
Fiber: 2g
Net Carbs: 1g
Protein: 5g
Fat: 7g

These Roasted Pumpkin Seeds with Sea Salt are a delicious and diabetic•friendly snack. Pumpkin seeds are a great source of healthy fats, protein, and fiber, making them an excellent choice for those following a diabetic diet.

The simple preparation of tossing the seeds in olive oil and seasoning them with sea salt allows the natural nutty flavor of the pumpkin seeds to shine. The roasting process gives them a satisfying crunch, making them a perfect snack to enjoy on their own or as a topping for salads, yogurt, or other dishes.

These Roasted Pumpkin Seeds with Sea Salt are a nutrient•dense and low•carb snack option that can help manage blood sugar levels. Enjoy them as a healthy and satisfying treat as part of your diabetic•friendly diet.

107. Jicama Sticks with Lime and Chili Powder

Ingredient:

• 1 medium jicama, peeled and cut into 1/4•inch thick sticks
• 1 tbsp fresh lime juice
• 1/2 tsp chili powder
• 1/4 tsp salt

Instructions:

1. Peel the jicama and cut it into 1/4•inch thick sticks or matchsticks.

2. In a large bowl, toss the jicama sticks with the fresh lime juice, chili powder, and salt until the jicama is evenly coated.

3. Serve the jicama sticks immediately, or refrigerate for up to 4 hours before serving.

Nutritional Information (per serving, about 1/2 cup):
Calories: 35
Total Carbs: 8g
Fiber: 3g
Net Carbs: 5g
Protein: 1g
Fat: 0g

Jicama is a great vegetable choice for a diabetic diet after 50. It is low in carbs, high in fiber, and has a refreshing, crunchy texture. The combination of lime juice and chili powder adds a zesty and flavorful twist to the jicama sticks, making them a delicious and diabetic•friendly snack.

The lime juice provides a boost of vitamin C, while the chili powder adds a touch of heat and antioxidants. This simple recipe is easy to prepare and can be enjoyed as a healthy snack or side dish.

Jicama Sticks with Lime and Chili Powder are a great option for those following a diabetic diet after 50, as they are low in carbs, high in fiber, and provide a satisfying crunch. Enjoy these tasty and nutritious jicama sticks as part of your diabetic•friendly diet.

108. Protein•Packed Green Smoothie

Ingredient:

• 1 cup unsweetened almond milk
• 1 scoop vanilla protein powder (choose a low•carb, sugar•free option)
• 1 cup packed spinach or kale
• 1/2 cup frozen berries (such as blueberries or raspberries)
• 1 tbsp ground flaxseed
• 1 tbsp nut butter (such as almond or peanut butter)
• 1 tsp cinnamon
• Ice cubes (optional)

Instructions:

1. Add all the ingredients to a high•powered blender.

2. Blend on high speed until the mixture is smooth and creamy, about 1•2 minutes.

3. If the smoothie is too thick, add a splash of extra almond milk and blend again.

4. Pour the smoothie into a glass and enjoy immediately.

This green smoothie is packed with protein, fiber, healthy fats, and essential vitamins and minerals • all important for managing diabetes after 50. The protein powder helps keep you feeling full and satisfied, while the greens, berries, and nut butter provide a nutrient•dense boost.

The cinnamon adds a touch of sweetness without any added sugar. This smoothie is low in carbs and high in nutrients, making it an excellent choice for a diabetic•friendly breakfast or snack.

Feel free to adjust the ingredients to your taste preferences. You can also add a handful of ice cubes to make the smoothie extra cold and refreshing.

Enjoy this delicious and nutritious protein•packed green smoothie as part of a balanced diabetic diet after 50!

1O9. Dill Pickles

Ingredient:

- 4 lbs pickling cucumbers, washed and cut into spears or chips
- 4 cups white vinegar
- 2 cups water
- 1/4 cup kosher salt
- 4 garlic cloves, peeled
- 4 sprigs fresh dill
- 2 tsp dill seeds
- 1 tsp black peppercorns

Instructions:

1. In a large pot, combine the vinegar, water, and salt. Bring to a boil, stirring to dissolve the salt. Remove from heat and let cool completely.

2. Pack the cucumber spears or chips tightly into 4 clean, quart·sized mason jars. Divide the garlic, dill sprigs, dill seeds, and peppercorns evenly between the jars.

3. Pour the cooled brine over the cucumbers, making sure they are fully submerged. Seal the jars.

4. Refrigerate for at least 2 weeks before eating. The pickles will keep in the refrigerator for up to 6 months.

That's it! The key is using fresh, crisp cucumbers and letting the pickles ferment for at least 2 weeks in the refrigerator brine. Enjoy your homemade dill pickles!

110. Zucchini Chips

Ingredient:
• 2 medium zucchinis, sliced into 1/8•inch thick rounds
• 1 tbsp olive oil
• 1/2 tsp garlic powder
• 1/2 tsp onion powder
• 1/4 tsp salt
• 1/4 tsp black pepper

Instructions:
1. Preheat your oven to 225°F (110°C). Line two baking sheets with parchment paper.

2. In a large bowl, toss the zucchini slices with the olive oil, garlic powder, onion powder, salt, and black pepper until the slices are evenly coated.

3. Arrange the zucchini slices in a single layer on the prepared baking sheets, making sure they are not overlapping.

4. Bake for 1 to 1 1/2 hours, flipping the zucchini slices halfway through, until they are crispy and lightly browned.

5. Remove the zucchini chips from the oven and let them cool completely on the baking sheets before serving.

Nutritional Information (per serving, about 10 chips):
Calories: 35
Total Carbs: 3g
Fiber: 1g
Net Carbs: 2g
Protein: 1g

These Zucchini Chips are a delicious and diabetic•friendly snack option. Zucchini is a low•carb vegetable that is high in fiber and nutrients, making it an excellent choice for those following a diabetic diet.

The baking process dehydrates the zucchini slices, creating a crispy and satisfying chip•like texture. The simple seasoning of garlic powder, onion powder, salt, and pepper adds flavor without adding too many additional carbs or calories.

These Zucchini Chips are a great alternative to traditional potato chips, providing a crunchy and satisfying snack that won't spike your blood sugar levels. Enjoy them on their own or with a dip of your choice for a diabetic•friendly treat.

111. Tofu Scramble with Spinach and Tomatoes

Ingredient:

- 1 block (14 oz) extra•firm tofu, drained and crumbled
- 1 tbsp olive oil
- 1 cup fresh spinach, chopped
- 1 cup cherry tomatoes, halved
- 1/2 tsp garlic powder
- 1/2 tsp onion powder
- 1/4 tsp turmeric
- 1/4 tsp black pepper
- 1/4 tsp salt (or to taste)

Instructions:

1. In a large non•stick skillet, heat the olive oil over medium heat.

2. Add the crumbled tofu and sauté for 2•3 minutes, breaking it up with a spatula as it cooks.

3. Stir in the spinach, cherry tomatoes, garlic powder, onion powder, turmeric, black pepper and salt. Cook for 3•4 minutes, stirring frequently, until the spinach is wilted and the tomatoes are slightly softened.

4. Taste and adjust seasoning as needed.

5. Serve hot, garnished with extra black pepper if desired.

This tofu scramble is high in protein, low in carbs, and packed with nutrient•dense vegetables • making it an excellent diabetic•friendly breakfast or brunch option. The combination of tofu, spinach and tomatoes provides fiber, vitamins and minerals important for managing diabetes after age 50.

112. Coconut Flour Pancakes

Ingredient:

• 1/2 cup coconut flour
• 2 eggs
• 1/4 cup unsweetened almond milk (or other non•dairy milk)
• 1 tsp baking powder
• 1/4 tsp salt
• 1 tsp vanilla extract (optional)
• 1•2 tbsp granulated erythritol or stevia (optional, to taste)

Instructions:

1. In a medium bowl, whisk together the coconut flour, eggs, almond milk, baking powder, salt, and vanilla (if using). Let the batter sit for 2•3 minutes to thicken.

2. If using a sweetener, stir it in now.

3. Heat a non•stick skillet or griddle over medium heat. Lightly grease with a small amount of oil or non•stick cooking spray.

4. Scoop the batter onto the hot surface, using about 2•3 tablespoons per pancake.

5. Cook for 2•3 minutes per side, until lightly golden brown. Flip carefully.

6. Serve the coconut flour pancakes warm, with your desired toppings such as fresh berries, a drizzle of sugar•free maple syrup, or a sprinkle of cinnamon.

These coconut flour pancakes are low in carbs, high in fiber and protein, making them an excellent choice for a diabetic•friendly breakfast. The coconut flour provides a light, fluffy texture. Feel free to adjust the sweetener to your taste preference.

113. Smoothie Bowl with Berries and Nuts

Ingredient:

- 1 cup frozen mixed berries (such as blueberries, raspberries, and blackberries)
- 1/2 cup unsweetened almond milk
- 1/2 cup plain Greek yogurt
- 1 tbsp ground flaxseeds
- 1 tbsp chopped walnuts or almonds
- 1 tsp honey (optional)

Instructions:

1. In a high·speed blender, combine the frozen mixed berries, almond milk, and Greek yogurt. Blend until smooth and creamy.

2. Pour the smoothie into a bowl.

3. Sprinkle the ground flaxseeds and chopped nuts over the top of the smoothie.

4. If desired, drizzle the honey over the top of the smoothie bowl.

Nutritional Information (per serving):
Calories: 250
Total Carbs: 22g
Fiber: 7g
Net Carbs: 15g
Protein: 15g
Fat: 12g

This Smoothie Bowl with Berries and Nuts is a delicious and diabetic·friendly breakfast or snack option. The combination of frozen berries, Greek yogurt, and almond milk provides a nutrient·dense and low·glycemic base.

The ground flaxseeds and chopped nuts add healthy fats, fiber, and additional nutrients to help keep you feeling full and satisfied. The optional honey can provide a touch of sweetness, but it can be omitted if you prefer a less sweet version.

This smoothie bowl is easy to prepare and can be customized to your taste preferences. It's a great way to incorporate more nutrient·dense foods into your diabetic·friendly diet.

Enjoy this Smoothie Bowl with Berries and Nuts as a delicious and healthy breakfast or snack!

114. Veggie and Cheese Breakfast Quesadilla

Ingredient:

• 2 low•carb whole wheat tortillas or high•fiber tortillas
• 1/2 cup shredded cheddar or Monterey Jack cheese
• 1/2 cup diced bell peppers
• 1/4 cup diced onions
• 1/4 cup diced tomatoes
• 2 eggs, scrambled
• 1 tbsp olive oil
• Salt and pepper to taste

Instructions:

1. In a small skillet, heat the olive oil over medium heat. Add the diced bell peppers and onions. Sauté for 3•4 minutes until softened.

2. Add the diced tomatoes and continue cooking for 1•2 minutes. Season with a pinch of salt and pepper.

3. In a separate pan, scramble the eggs until cooked through.

4. Place one tortilla in a clean skillet or griddle over medium heat. Top half of the tortilla with half of the shredded cheese, followed by the sautéed veggies and scrambled eggs.

5. Fold the other half of the tortilla over the filling to create a half•moon shape. Cook for 2•3 minutes per side, until the tortilla is lightly golden and the cheese is melted.

6. Repeat with the remaining tortilla, veggies and eggs to make a second quesadilla.

7. Slice each quesadilla in half and serve warm.

This breakfast quesadilla is packed with fiber, protein and nutrients from the veggies, making it a great diabetic•friendly option. The whole wheat or high•fiber tortilla helps keep the carbs in check.

115. Berry and Almond Butter Smoothie

Ingredient:

- 1 cup unsweetened almond milk
- 1/2 cup frozen mixed berries (such as raspberries, blueberries, strawberries)
- 2 tbsp natural almond butter
- 1 tbsp ground flaxseed
- 1 tsp vanilla extract
- 1/4 tsp cinnamon
- 1•2 tsp granulated erythritol or stevia (optional, to taste)

Instructions:

1. Add all the ingredients to a high•powered blender.

2. Blend on high speed until the mixture is smooth and creamy, about 1 minute.

3. Taste and adjust sweetener if desired. The berries provide natural sweetness, but you can add a bit of erythritol or stevia if you prefer it sweeter.

4. Pour the smoothie into a glass and enjoy immediately.

This smoothie is a great diabetic•friendly breakfast or snack option. The combination of almond milk, almond butter, berries, and flaxseed provides a balance of protein, healthy fats, fiber, and complex carbs to help manage blood sugar levels.

The cinnamon also helps regulate blood sugar. Feel free to adjust the ingredient amounts to suit your personal taste preferences. You can also add a handful of spinach or kale for an extra nutrient boost.

116. Egg White and Spinach Wrap

Ingredient:

• 2 large egg whites
• 1/2 cup fresh spinach, chopped
• 1 tbsp diced onion
• 1 tbsp diced bell pepper
• 1 tbsp shredded cheddar cheese
• 1 low•carb or high•fiber tortilla wrap
• Salt and pepper to taste

Instructions:

1. In a small non•stick skillet, lightly coat with cooking spray and heat over medium heat.

2. Add the diced onion and bell pepper. Sauté for 2•3 minutes until softened.

3. Pour in the egg whites and let them cook for 1•2 minutes, then use a spatula to gently scramble the eggs.

4. Once the eggs are mostly cooked through, add the chopped spinach and continue cooking for another 1•2 minutes, until the spinach is wilted.

5. Season the egg mixture with a pinch of salt and pepper.

6. Lay the tortilla wrap on a flat surface. Spoon the egg white and veggie mixture onto the center of the wrap.

7. Sprinkle the shredded cheddar cheese over the top.

8. Fold the bottom of the wrap up over the filling, then fold in the sides and continue rolling up tightly.

9. Serve the egg white and spinach wrap warm.

This wrap is high in protein from the egg whites, and packed with nutrient•dense vegetables. The low•carb tortilla helps keep the carb count in check, making it a great diabetic•friendly breakfast option.

117. Low•Carb Banana Pancakes

Ingredient:

• 2 ripe bananas, mashed
• 3 eggs
• 1/4 cup almond flour
• 1 tsp baking powder
• 1/4 tsp cinnamon
• 1/4 tsp vanilla extract
• Pinch of salt

Instructions:

1. In a medium bowl, mash the ripe bananas until smooth.

2. Add the eggs and whisk together until well combined.

3. Stir in the almond flour, baking powder, cinnamon, vanilla, and salt. Mix until a smooth batter forms.

4. Heat a lightly oiled non•stick skillet or griddle over medium heat.

5. Scoop the batter onto the hot surface, using about 1/4 cup per pancake.

6. Cook for 2•3 minutes per side, until golden brown.

7. Serve the low•carb banana pancakes warm, with your favorite toppings like berries, nuts, or sugar•free syrup.

These pancakes are gluten•free, low in carbs, and get their sweetness from the ripe bananas. Enjoy this healthier take on classic banana pancakes!

*As you reach the end of **"Diabetic Diet Cookbook After 50: 115+ A Culinary Guide to Managing Diabetes and Aging Gracefully,"** we hope you feel empowered and inspired to continue your journey toward a healthier and more vibrant life. This book was designed to provide you with practical tools and delicious recipes that make managing diabetes both enjoyable and sustainable.*

Embracing a diabetic-friendly diet after 50 is more than just a necessity; it's an opportunity to explore new flavors, ingredients, and culinary techniques. The recipes in this book are tailored to meet your nutritional needs while ensuring that every meal is satisfying and delightful. From hearty breakfasts to satisfying dinners, and everything in between, you now have a robust collection of dishes to keep your palate excited and your blood sugar levels in check.

Beyond the recipes, we have also shared essential tips and insights to help you navigate your diabetic diet with confidence. Understanding how to plan your meals, shop smartly, and balance your diet with physical activity and stress management are crucial steps in maintaining your health and well-being.

Remember, managing diabetes is a lifelong journey that requires commitment, but it is also a journey that can be filled with joy, discovery, and satisfaction. By choosing to nourish your body with wholesome, balanced meals, you are taking a proactive step towards better health and a higher quality of life.

We encourage you to revisit these recipes often, experiment with new ingredients, and make cooking an enjoyable part of your daily routine. Share these meals with loved ones and embrace the communal aspect of eating well.

Thank you for allowing us to be a part of your health journey. May this cookbook continue to serve as a valuable resource and a source of inspiration as you age gracefully and manage your diabetes with confidence and creativity.

Here's to your health, happiness, and many delicious meals ahead!